Summer Fresh Salads 2021

Your new, easy recipes for a healthy summer

Nicole Forest

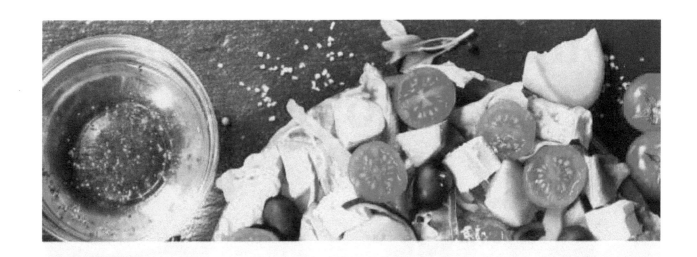

SUMMER FRESH SALADS
2021

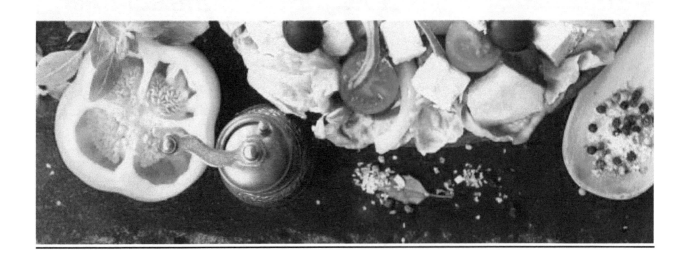

Sommario

INTRODUCTION 6

1. Gift salad 7
2. Salad "Sea King" 9
3. Cod liver salad 11
4. Shrimp and curd cheese salad 13
5. beetroot salad with chicken 15
6. Combined salad with tomatoes and ham 17
7. A nutritious protein salad: sheer pleasure! 19
8. Delicious salad with chicken and prunes 21
9. Chicken and omelet salad 23
10. "Your" salad 25
11. Bean salad 27
12. English salad, be sure to try it! 29
13. Layered salad "Pearl" 31
14. Delicious salad for the festive table! 33
15. SEA SALATIC 35
16. Tuna salad with corn for dinner! 37
17. Chicken salad "Bunch of grapes" 39
18. Chicken and apple salad 41
19. Italian salad with ham, cheese and vegetables 43
20. Salad "Dubok" 45
21. Red Sea salad 47
22. Very original Negresco salad 49
23. "Flagman" salad 51
24. Curd salad for losing weight. 53
25. Chicken salad with carrots and green peas 250 g of boiled chicken meat, ... 55
26. Delicious salad for the festive table. 57
27. Coleslaw salad. 59
28. Fresh vegetable salad with beef 61
29. Amazing crab salad. 63
30. Chicken and prune salad for dinner 65
31. Salad with chicken breast, tomatoes and green peas. 67
32. "Bride" salad. 69
33. Tomato salad with boiled smoked brisket, cheese and croutons. 71
34. Festive Cod Liver Salad. 73
35. Delicious salad with herring 75
36. Delicious vinaigrette 77
37. Bean salad for dinner! 79
38. Low-calorie "Protein" salad 81
39. Chicken fillet salad with green beans 83
40. Simple and hearty salad 85
41. Chicken breast and corn salad. 87
42. Cole Slow Diet Salad 89
43. Fresh cabbage salad with chicken 91

44.   Beetroot salad: the right yummy!... 93

45.   Salat "Emerald" 95

46.   Baked salmon with mushrooms 97

47.   Venice salad 100

48.   Egg and ham salad.. 102

49.   Layered salad "my general" 104

INTRODUCTION

Welcome to the salad cookbook, designed to completely change your relationship with fruits and vegetables.

When it comes to salads, simple tricks can make a big impact on flavor and enjoyment. Many of the salads in this book are inspired by flavors from cuisines around the world.

These diverse and highly versatile recipes make for perfect side dishes or starters, and many of them can also stand alone as healthy meals. Along with 49 salad recipes, as well as tips for making salad prep fast and easy.

Great salads shouldn't be reserved for the dinner table. Many recipes in this book also include a make-and-take layering technique for packing salads to go, so you can eat them for lunch wherever you are, from the office to the park to the gym.

Enjoy seeing—and eating—salads in a whole new light!

1. GIFT SALAD

Ingredients:

- smoked chicken breast 300g

- champignons 300g

- onion 1pc.

- pickled cucumbers 3pcs.

- carrots 1pc.

- eggs 4pcs.

- fresh pepper 1pc. (large)

- fresh cucumber for decoration

- mayonnaise 250

Preparation:

Cut the breast, pickled cucumbers into cubes. Fry the champignons with onions, salt and pepper. Boil carrots and eggs, grate on a coarse grater. Finely chop the pepper. Put the salad in layers in a 21cm ring, coat the layers with mayonnaise.

Layers:

- smoked chicken breast

- pickled cucumbers

- carrot

- eggs

- champignons with onions

- pepper

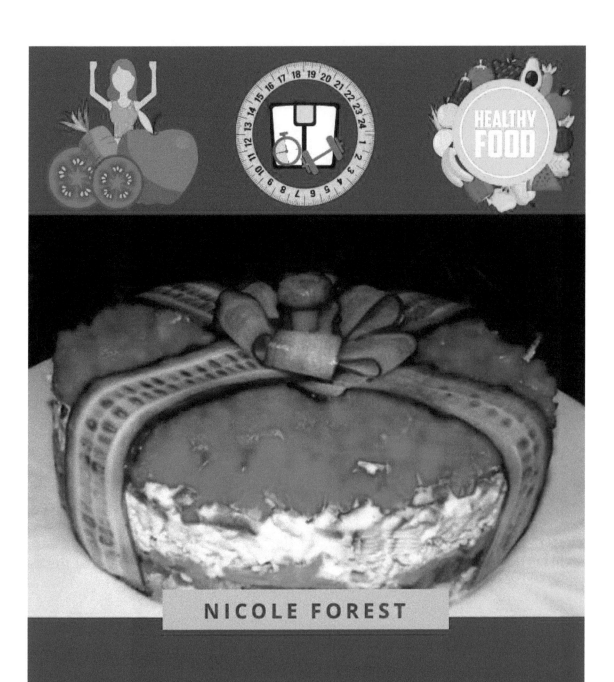

NICOLE FOREST

Gift Salad

2. SALAD "SEA KING"

Ingredients
Frozen squids - 800 g. Fillet
of sea fish - 400 g. Onions - 1
pc.
Carrots - 2 pcs.
Eggs - 4 pcs.
White cabbage - 300 g.
Mayonnaise - 350 g.
Salt to taste.

Cooking method

Step 1 Boil the squid in salted water from the moment the water boils for 4 minutes, cool, peel, cut into strips.

Step 2 Boil the carrots, peel and cut into cubes. Step 3
Boil the eggs, cool, peel and cut into cubes.
Step 4 Chop the cabbage, salt and rub well with your hands. Step
5 Finely chop the onion, fry until golden brown, add to the onion fish
fillet cut into pieces, fry until fish is ready, add salt,
cool, drain excess oil (you can use a sieve).

Step 6 Mix all the ingredients, season with mayonnaise.

Step 7 Decorate the salad with egg whites, lingonberries, and parsley leaves. Enjoy your meal!

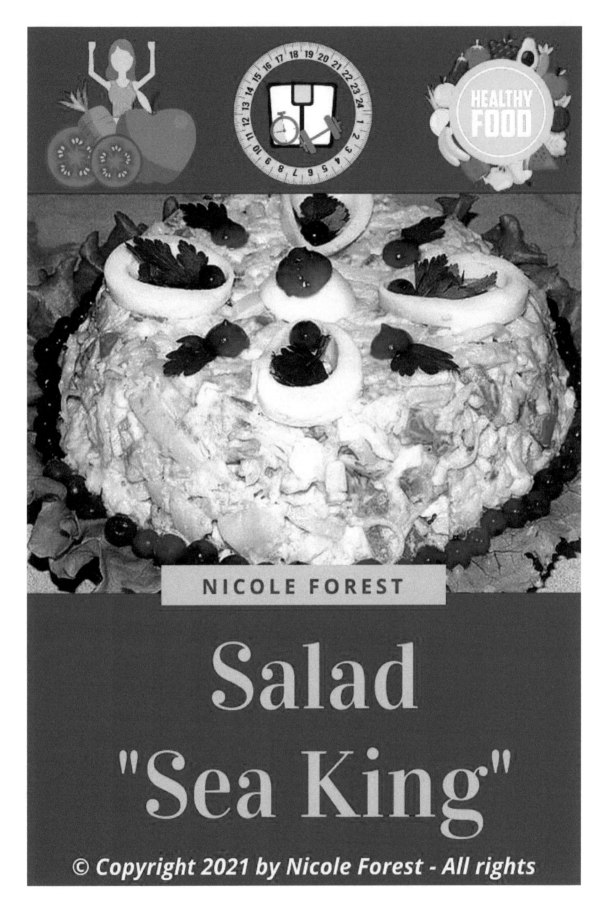

NICOLE FOREST

Salad
"Sea King"

3. COD LIVER SALAD

Cod liver is the main source of such a useful and irreplaceable product as fish oil. It contains a large amount of vitamins A and D. I want to share a recipe for cod liver salad, it turns out to be tender and tasty, and the addition of pickled cucumber gives the dish a special piquancy.

To prepare the salad you will need: cod
liver - 1 can;
egg - 2 pcs.;
peas - 1/2 can;
pickled cucumber - 2-3 pcs. (small);
green onion;

mayonnaise - 1 tbsp. l.

Prepare foods for the salad. Hard-boiled eggs, cool and peel. Remove the cod liver from the jar and drain off the excess oil. Wash and dry the onion. Drain the liquid from the peas.

Cut the cucumbers into cubes. Finely chop the onion, liver, eggs. Combine cod liver, eggs, peas, onions, cucumber, mayonnaise. Mix the salad well.

This cod liver salad can be served in a salad bowl, or you can do it in portions.

Enjoy your meal!

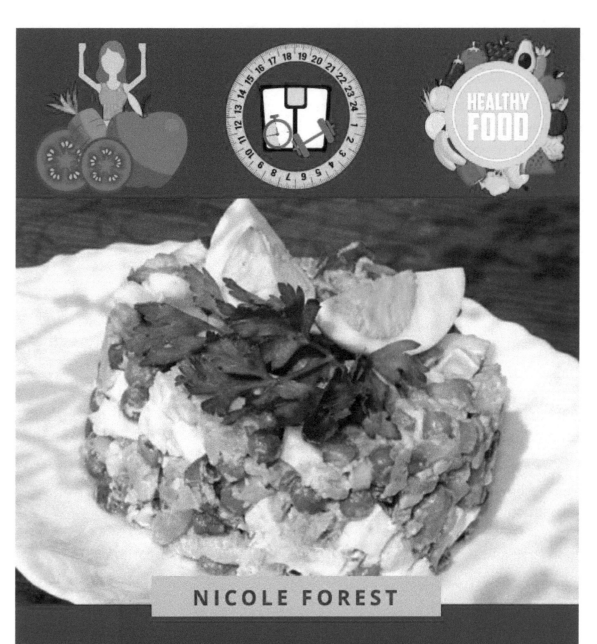

NICOLE FOREST

Cod liver salad

4. **SHRIMP AND CURD CHEESE SALAD**

Ingredients:

shrimp (large) 180 g (boiled and peeled from the shell) 1/4
lemon juice
fresh greens 20 g
cucumber 120 g
low-fat curd cheese 100 g 1
clove garlic
salt and pepper to taste

Preparation:

Boil the shrimps in salted water, peel off the shell. Chop shrimp and drizzle with lemon juice

Cut the peel from the cucumber, cut into cubes, chop the herbs.

Combine chopped shrimp, cucumber, herbs and garlic squeezed through a garlic press.

Add curd cheese, mix well, pepper if desired.

You can serve in tartlets or make portions using the culinary ring, I put it on lettuce leaves, and sprinkle with herbs

Enjoy your meal!

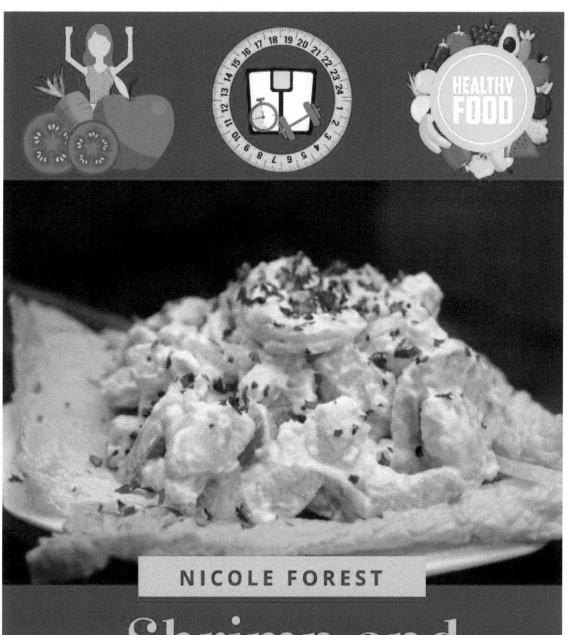

NICOLE FOREST

Shrimp and curd cheese salad

5. BEETROOT SALAD WITH CHICKEN

Ingredients:

Beets 4 pcs. (400 g) Boiled
chicken fillet 400 g Walnuts
0.5 cups
Natural yogurt 0.5 cups
Greenery for decoration
Salt, pepper to taste

Preparation:

Fry the walnuts in a dry frying pan for a couple of minutes. Dice the
beets and chicken breast. Chop the nuts.
Mix all the ingredients, season with yogurt and salt - pepper to taste.

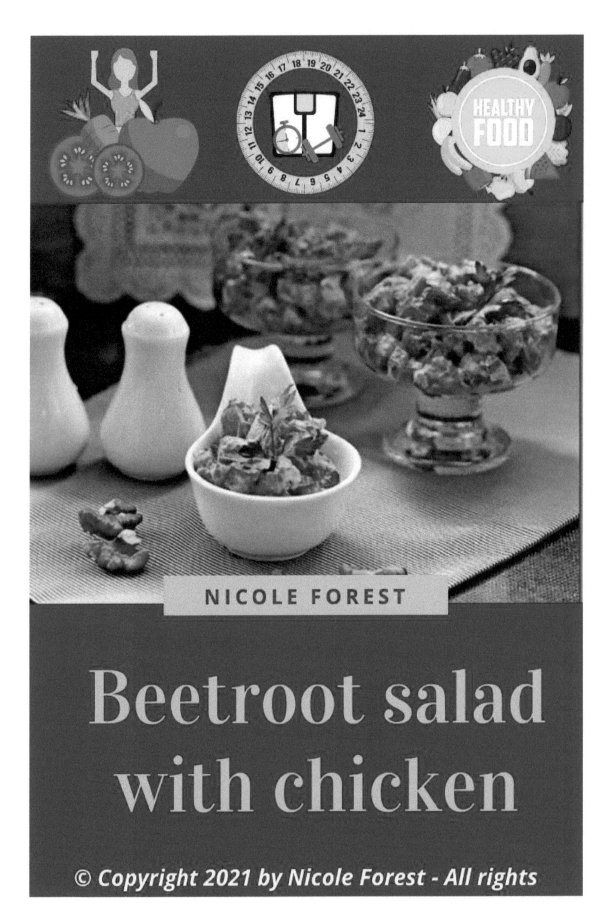

HEALTHY FOOD

NICOLE FOREST

Beetroot salad with chicken

6. COMBINED SALAD WITH TOMATOES AND HAM

Ingredients:
-Tomatoes - 300 gr.

-Ham - 200 gr.

-Green peas - 1 can

-Cheese - 150 gr.

-Salt

-Mayonnaise

Preparation:

Tomatoes, ham - cubed. Drain
the juice from the peas. Cheese
on a coarse grater.
Season with salt, season with mayonnaise.
Notes:

* When the salad is exactly in the form I have now, it will be very tasty to add garlic (garlic press) and 100 grams of croutons.

* Instead of peas, you can take a couple of small cucumbers.

* Canned beans can be used instead of peas.

* If instead of peas there are cucumbers, then it will also be delicious instead of tomatoes to take Bulgarian pepper.

* You can add chopped herbs (onions, dill, parsley - to taste) Enjoy your meal!

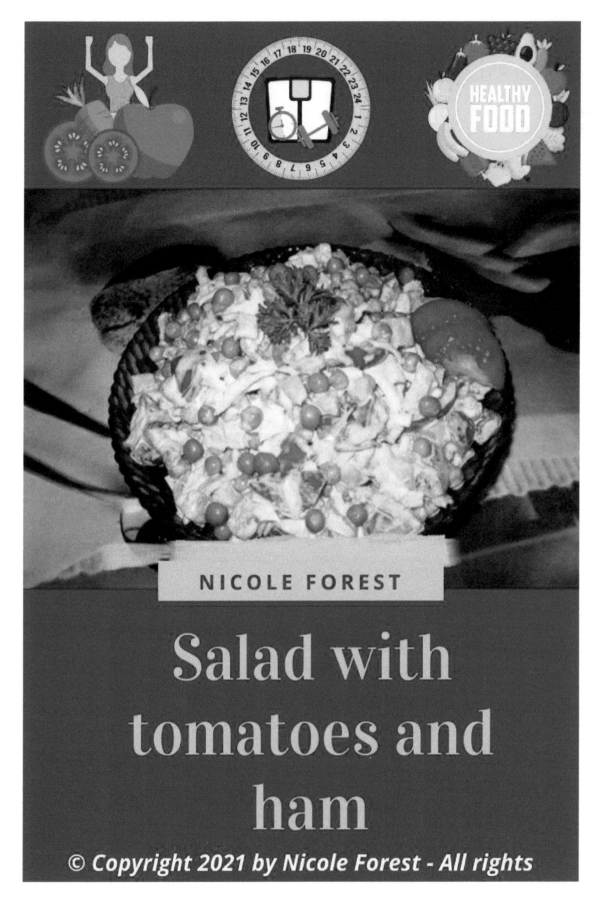

NICOLE FOREST

Salad with tomatoes and ham

7. A NUTRITIOUS PROTEIN SALAD: SHEER PLEASURE!

Ingredients:

Canned beans - 1/2 can
Proteins - 3 pcs (boiled)
Yolks - 2 pcs (boiled)
Cucumber - 1 pc (salted)

Greens to taste
Onions to taste

For refueling:

Natural yogurt - 3 tbsp l
Mustard - 1 tsp

Preparation:

Cut the whites, yolks, cucumber into squares. Chop the greens and onions and drain
the beans.

Combine and season all ingredients. dressing, mix. Enjoy
your meal!

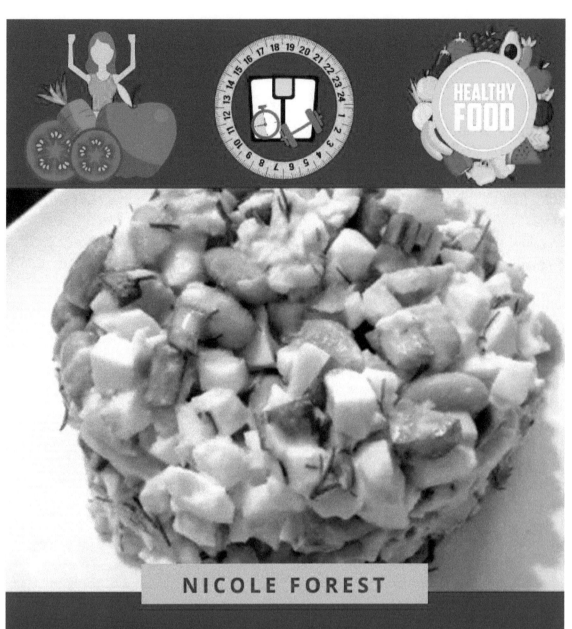

NICOLE FOREST

A nutritious protein salad: sheer pleasure!

8. DELICIOUS SALAD WITH CHICKEN AND PRUNES

Ingredients:

400gr. white chicken meat,
100gr. prunes,
1 carrot,

2 tbsp canned corn

100gr. sour cream,

2 tbsp olives (pitted),
Salt to taste

Preparation:

Cut the meat (if desired, I made cubes). Soak the prunes in water, then cut them. Grate the carrots on a coarse grater. Mix everything, Add corn, olives. Season with salt and sour cream. Decorate to taste.

Enjoy your meal!

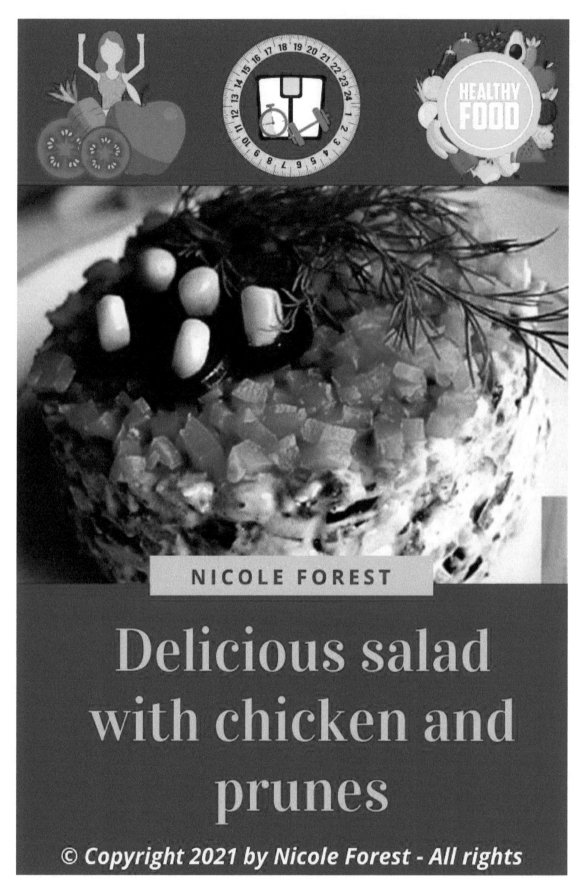

NICOLE FOREST

Delicious salad with chicken and prunes

9. <u>CHICKEN AND OMELET SALAD</u>

Ingredients:

1 chicken fillet

4 fresh cucumbers

1 fresh carrot

For the omelet:

1 egg

1 tbsp milk

1 pinch of salt
For refueling:

2 cloves of garlic 1
tbsp soy sauce 1
tbsp olive oil
1 tsp vinegar

Boil fillets until tender, cut into strips, also cut cucumbers and carrots

Beat the egg with milk and salt, prepare a thin omelet in a non-stick frying pan, greased with a drop of oil.

Let it cool, also cut into strips

Combine the ingredients for the dressing, except for the garlic, stir, beat lightly, then add the garlic passed through a press.

Enjoy your meal!

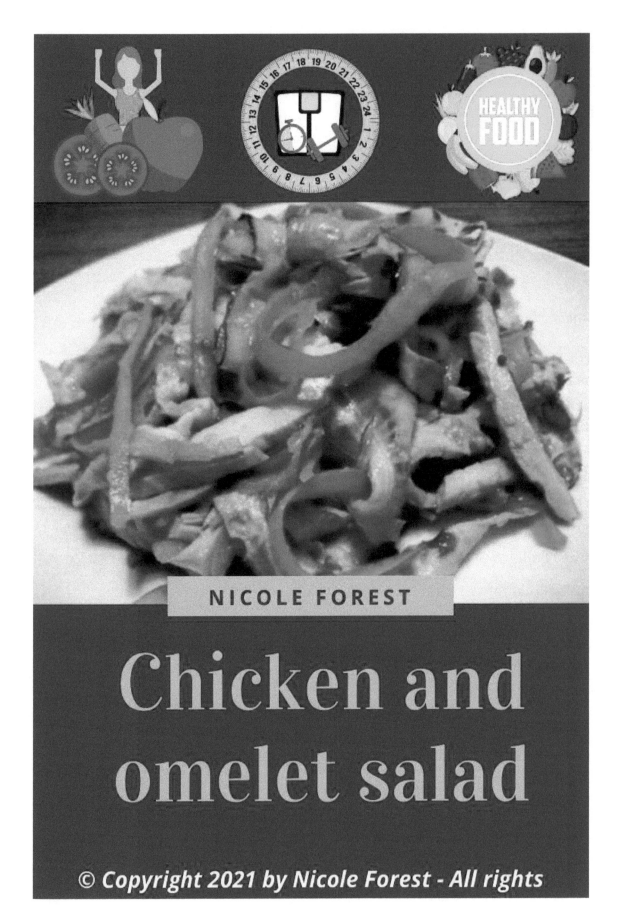

NICOLE FOREST

Chicken and omelet salad

10.   "YOUR" SALAD

The recipe was sent to us by a member of our page

Ingredients:

-Chicken fillet 150-200 gr

-Ham 150 gr

-Fresh tomatoes 250g

- Croutons 100 gr

-Mayonnaise 200gr

-Adzhika 15gr

-Garlic 10 gr

-Vegetable oil for frying

Preparation:

cut all the ingredients into the same block. Fry raw chicken until tender, you can add a pinch of chicken seasoning. I cooked with seasoning, it gives a beautiful golden color. Season with salt at the end of frying. Fry the ham in a hot frying pan until golden brown. Put rye-wheat bread on a baking sheet, salt and pour with a small amount of vegetable oil, no more than a teaspoon. We put in the oven preheated to 250 degrees, dry until lightly browning.
Tomatoes stay fresh. We put everything on a flat plate in layers. I put the fried fillet first, then half the tomato so that the chicken is soaked in juice, the next layer is the fried ham, coat everything with mayonnaise + adjika + garlic dressing, then lay out the rest of the tomato. Top before serving with a slide of croutons.

The salad turns out to be unusual, quite satisfying, moderately spicy and aromatic. Your guests will be satisfied

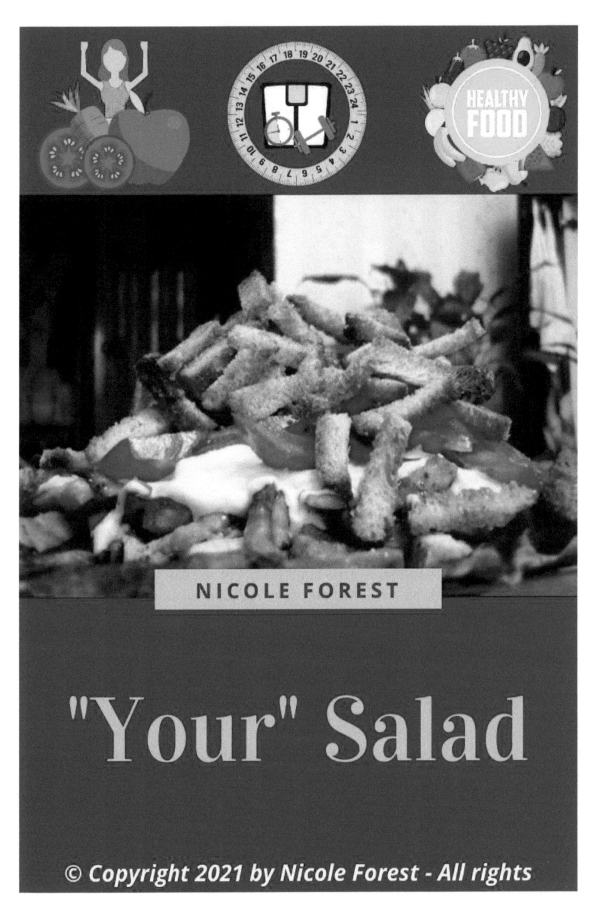

NICOLE FOREST

"Your" Salad

11. BEAN SALAD

Ingredients:
- Tomato 2-3 pcs.

- Chicken breast 500gr.

- Hard cheese 150 gr.

- Red beans - one can.

- Green salad.

- Crackers.

- For dressing, you can take light mayonnaise or sour cream.

Preparation:

1. Finely chop the tomato, lettuce. Three cheese on a grater.

2. Cut the chicken breast into small pieces and simmer over low heat for about 20 minutes until all the liquid boils away, you can lightly fry.

3. Mix all the chopped and ready-made ingredients, season with mayonnaise (sour cream). Serve the salad, sprinkle with croutons on top.

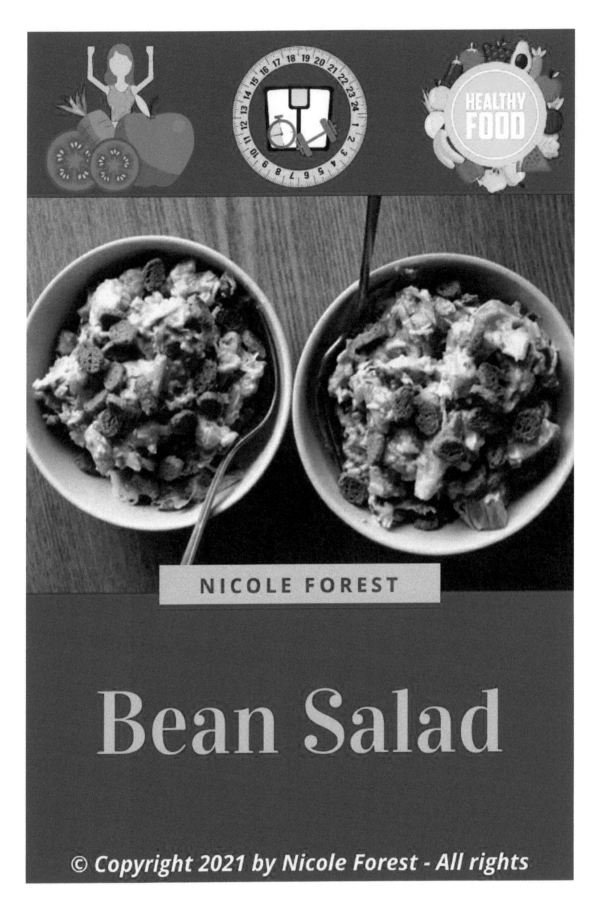

NICOLE FOREST

Bean Salad

12.   **ENGLISH SALAD, BE SURE TO TRY IT!**

Ingredients: Canned
corn 285 g
Chicken breast 1 piece

Champignons 500 g

Tomatoes 3 pieces

Croutons 100 g
Sour cream 150 g

Preparation:

1. Boil chicken breasts and chopped mushrooms. Chop finely and transfer to a bowl.

2. Add a can of corn.

3. Then add the croutons.

4. Stir in the finely chopped tomatoes.

5. Add sour cream and stir gently.

Enjoy your me

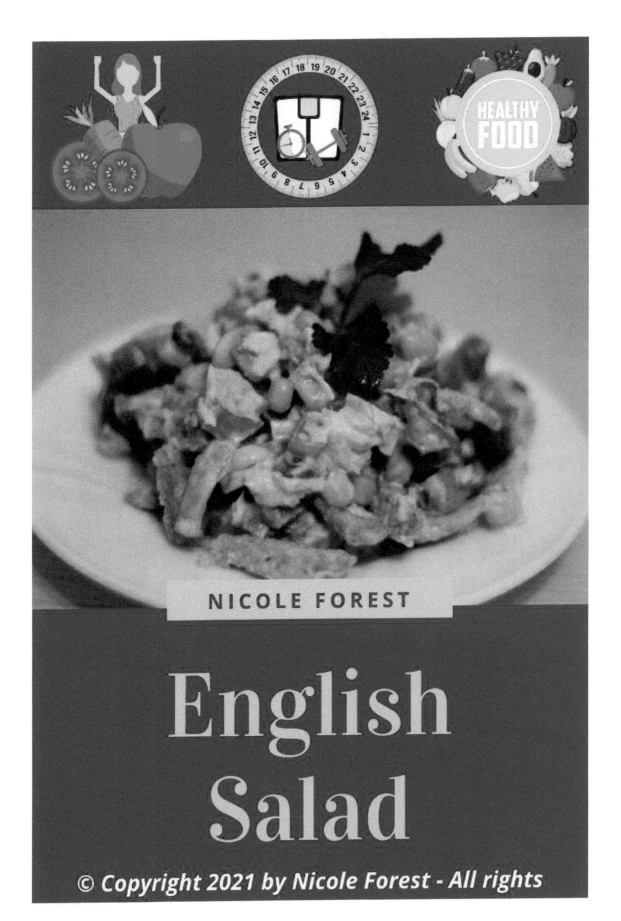

NICOLE FOREST

English Salad

13.   LAYERED SALAD "PEARL"

Ingredients:
200 g lightly salted salmon
40-50 g olives
60 g cheese

5 eggs

1 orange

1-2 tablespoons red caviar
mayonnaise
salt

pepper green
onions

Preparation:

Boil the eggs hard-boiled, separate the whites from the yolks and grate on a medium grater.

Cut the salmon into small slices.

Peel the orange peel and fibers and cut the flesh into cubes. Rub the cheese on a fine grater.
Cut the olives into rings. Lay out the salad in layers.
The first layer is half of the proteins mixed with mayonnaise.

Next, lay out the yolks, salt, pepper to taste and coat a little with mayonnaise. Spread half of the salmon with the third layer and coat with mayonnaise.
Then the olives and the rest of the salmon.

Then we spread the cheese and some mayonnaise.

Put oranges in the next layer, and on top of the remaining proteins mixed with mayonnaise.

Decorate the salad with caviar and olives, and put half a quail egg in the center.

Put the ready-made "Pearl" salad in the refrigerator, after wrapping it with cling film, and let it brew for several hours.

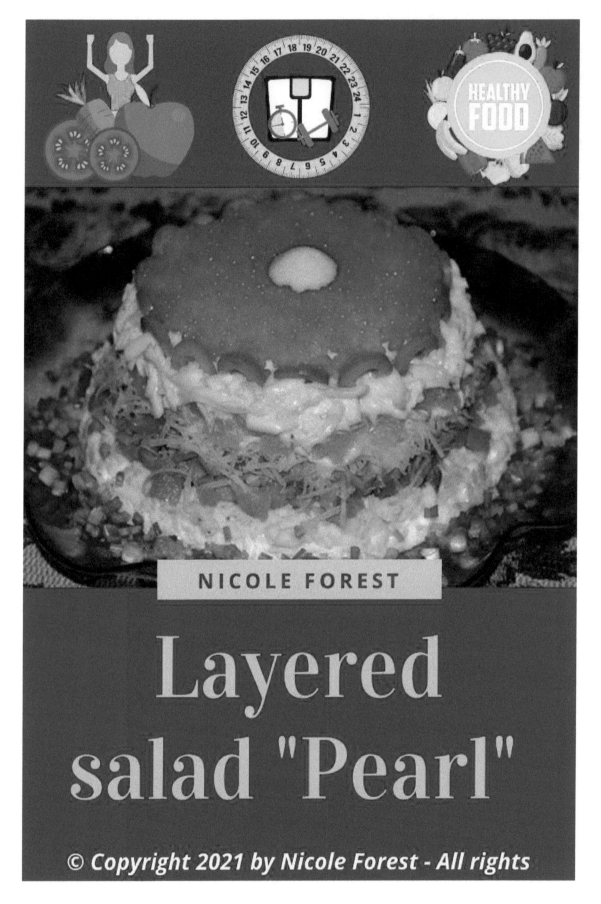

HEALTHY FOOD

NICOLE FOREST

Layered salad "Pearl"

14. DELICIOUS SALAD FOR THE FESTIVE TABLE!

Ingredients:

- Chicken breast-2 pcs (800gr),

- Champignons 600-700gr,

- 6 boiled eggs.

- 2-3 medium-sized onions,

- 2-3 medium carrots,

- hard cheese 100g,

- mayonnaise,

- spices (curry),

- greens.
Preparation:
Fry mushrooms with onions and put in a colander (so that excess fat is gone) Fry the breast with curry, cut into cubes. eggs (cut the yolks too) add mayonnaise, or sour cream, salt to taste. Put on a dish, giving the shape of a mushroom, decorate the leg with protein grated on a fine grater (sprinkle with dill), a hat-boiled carrots grated on a fine grater, the bottom of the cap with grated cheese.

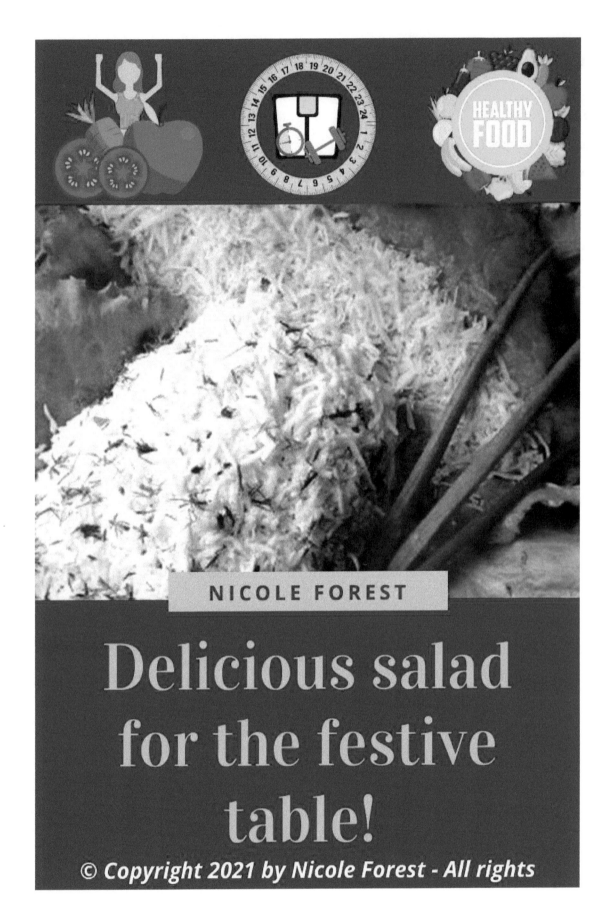

NICOLE FOREST

Delicious salad for the festive table!

15. SEA SALATIC

INGREDIENTS:

- 1 layer-crab meat

- 2 layer tomato

- 3 layer - cheese (grated),

- 4 layer cucumber,

- 5 layer - rice (boiled),

- 6 layer cheese,

COOKING:

In the reverse order, put everything in a mold (any) Spread each layer with mayonnaise. Let him lie down for 2 hours ..

Delight salad with squid, cucumber and carrots
Ingredients:

Squid - 300 g
Egg - 2 pieces
Carrots - 100 g
Fresh cucumber - 100 g
Petiole celery - 50 g
Natural yogurt - 50 g Salt,
pepper - to taste

Preparation:

Prepare the squid. Dip them in boiling water for 1 minute, then remove and clean under running cold water from all external and internal films. Cut the cooled boiled squid into strips.

Boil the carrots until tender for 20 minutes, cool and peel. Cut the peeled carrots into strips. Cut fresh cucumber into strips. Combine chopped squid, carrots and cucumbers in one bowl. Add finely chopped stalked celery and eggs. Season the squid salad with salt and pepper. Add yogurt and stir.
Transfer the squid, cucumber and carrot salad to a dish or bowl and serve. Enjoy your meal!

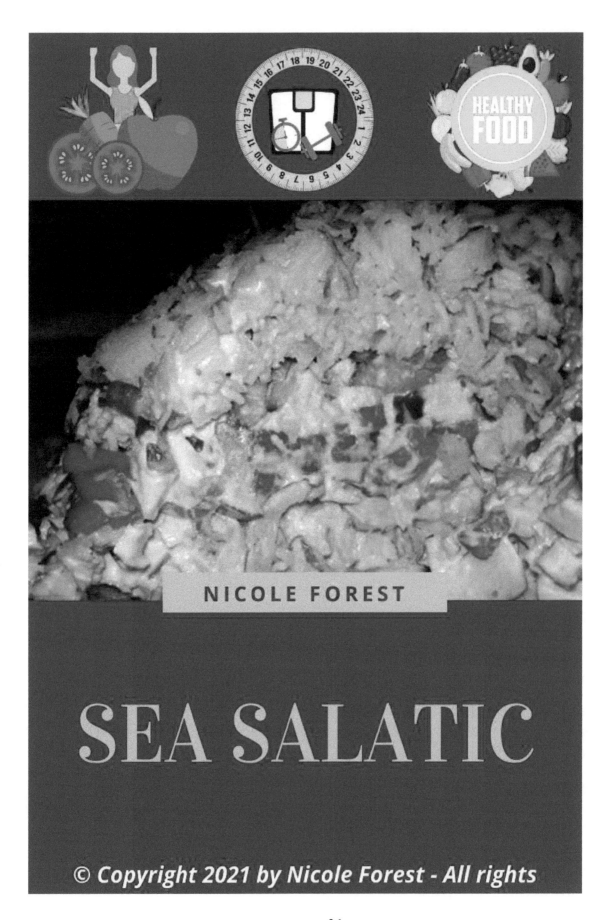

NICOLE FOREST

SEA SALATIC

16.   TUNA SALAD WITH CORN FOR DINNER!

Ingredients:

Canned tuna in its own juice 1 can
Pickled cucumbers 4 pcs
Canned corn 200 g

Onion 1 head
Chicken egg 4 pcs
Low-fat sour cream 100 g

Greens to taste
Salt to taste

Preparation:

1. Add finely grated onion to chopped fish and stir.

2. Boil hard-boiled eggs and grate on a coarse grater. ...

3. Peel the cucumbers, cut

4. Stir in egg, fish and onion, cucumber and corn. Season the salad with sour cream. Salt.

Enjoy your meal!

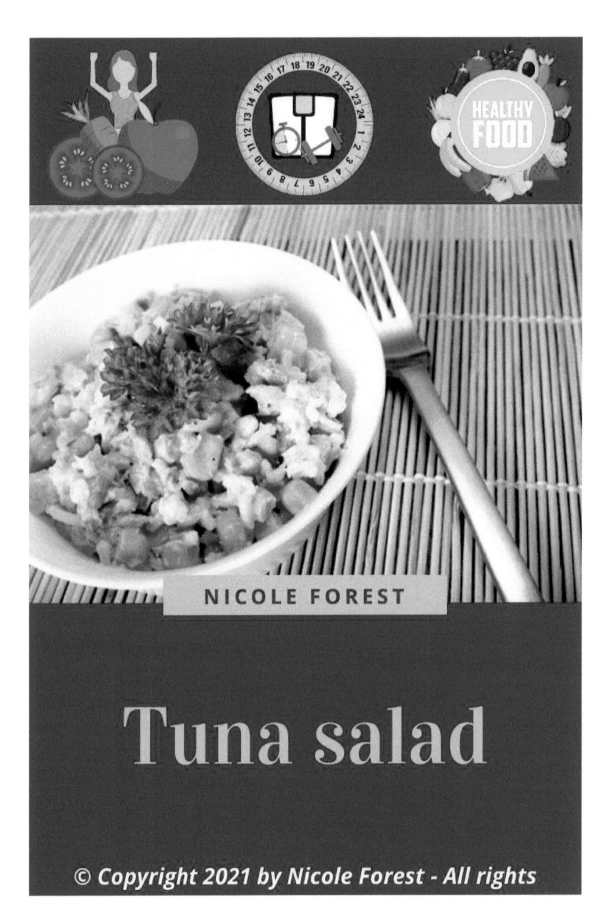

NICOLE FOREST

Tuna salad

17.CHICKEN SALAD "BUNCH OF GRAPES"

Ingredients:

-400 g smoked chicken fillet

-300 g of hard cheese

-300 g pitted dark grapes

-3 boiled eggs

-mayonnaise

-parsley

Preparation:

1. Spread the salad in layers: proteins, chicken fillet, yolks, cheese, smearing each layer with mayonnaise.

2. Place the grapes in a bunch and around the perimeter of the salad.

3. Before serving, garnish with herbs and refrigerate.

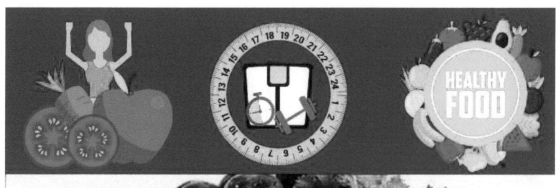

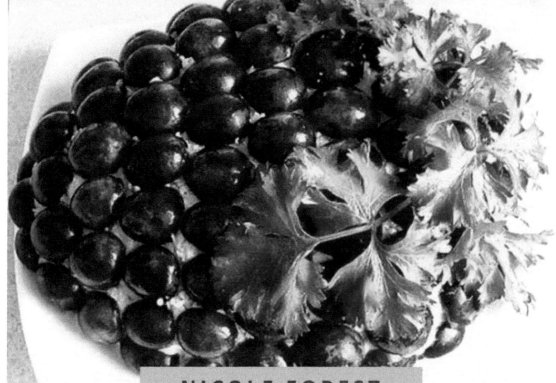

NICOLE FOREST

Chicken Salad

18.   CHICKEN AND APPLE SALAD

Ingredients:

Chicken breast (boiled) 1 pc.
Apple (sour) 1 pc.
Hard cheese 70g

Egg (protein) 4 pcs.
Natural yogurt 100ml a
handful of seeds
Mustard, salt and pepper to taste.

Preparation:

Chop up chicken breast, apples, eggs and cheese.

Dressing: Mix natural yogurt with mustard, salt and pepper, add a little lemon juice to taste. Season the chicken salad with the seeds and stir.

Enjoy your mea

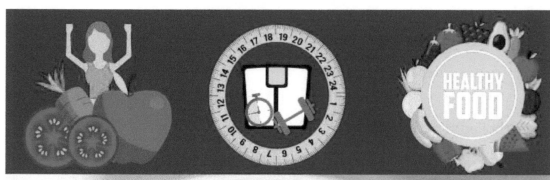

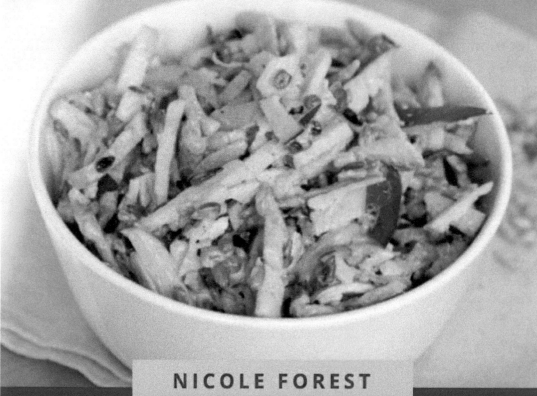

NICOLE FOREST

Chicken and apple salad

19. ITALIAN SALAD WITH HAM, CHEESE AND VEGETABLES

Ingredients:

- Ham - 300 g

- Pomidopes - 2 pieces

- Bolgar pepper - 2 pieces

- Macaroons - 400 g

- Canned corn - 300 g

- Cheese - 200 g

- Mayones - to taste

Preparation:

Open the macaroons - it is best to use pozhki or spiral macaroons - in hot water, drain and let them settle.

Cut the pots and peppers into cubes, the ham into thin slices. Wipe the cheese on a large block.

Mix all the ingredients, season the salad with mayonnaise.

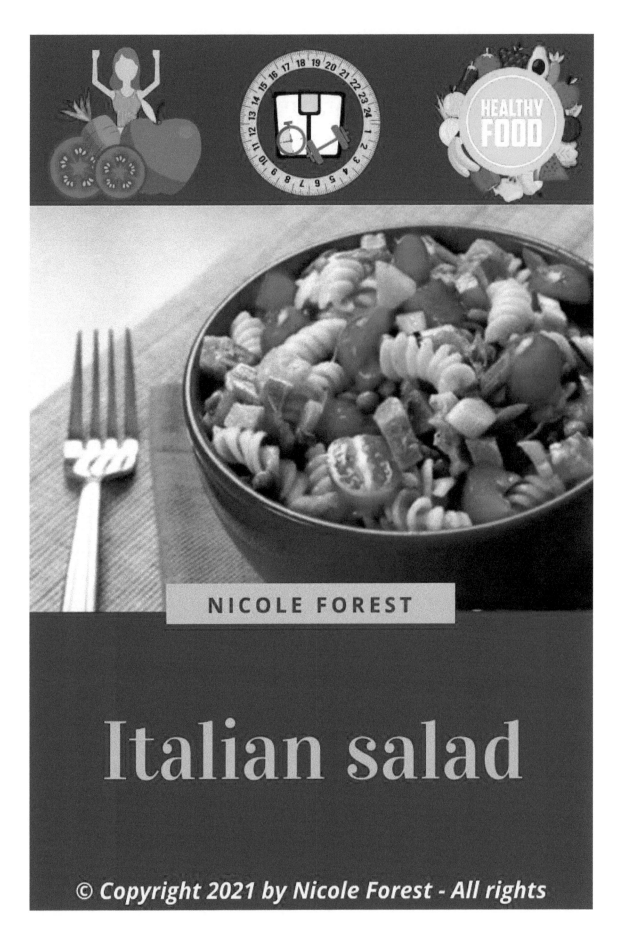

HEALTHY
FOOD

NICOLE FOREST

Italian salad

20. **<u>SALAD "DUBOK"</u>**

Ingredients:

2 medium boiled potatoes
1/2 chicken breast
1 pickled cucumber (can be substituted with salted) 1 can of canned mushrooms
1 egg

mayonnaise (for coating layers) dill
(for decoration)

Preparation:

Layer in layers on a flat dish:

potatoes (grate)
mayonnaise
chicken fillet (boil and chop finely)

mayonnaise

pickled cucumber (grate, if necessary, you can replace with salted) mayonnaise
champignons (squeeze the "brine", chop finely)
mayonnaise
egg (grate)
potatoes (grate)
mayonnaise
dill (finely chopped)

Leave on for 30 minutes. at room temperature (soak). Then refrigerate and serve.

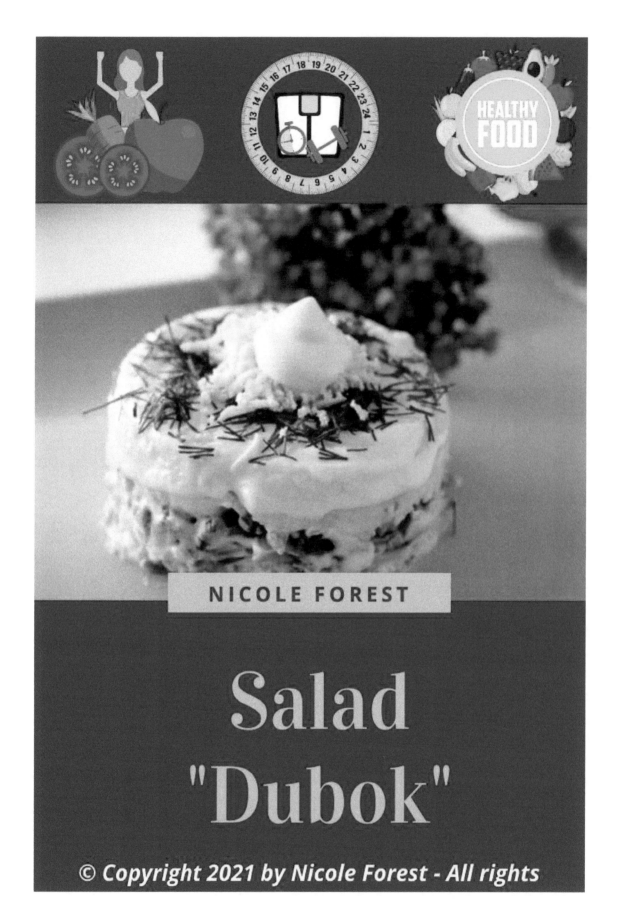

NICOLE FOREST

Salad "Dubok"

21.   **RED SEA SALAD**

Ingredients:
squid - 250-300 g
tomatoes - 1-2 pcs.
cheese - 100-200 g
garlic - 1 clove
mayonnaise

Preparation:

1. Peel and boil squids in salted water for 1-2 minutes. Cut into strips.

2. Cut the tomatoes into strips too.

3. Squeeze the garlic through a press. Grate cheese on a coarse grater.

4. Mix everything and season with mayonnaise.

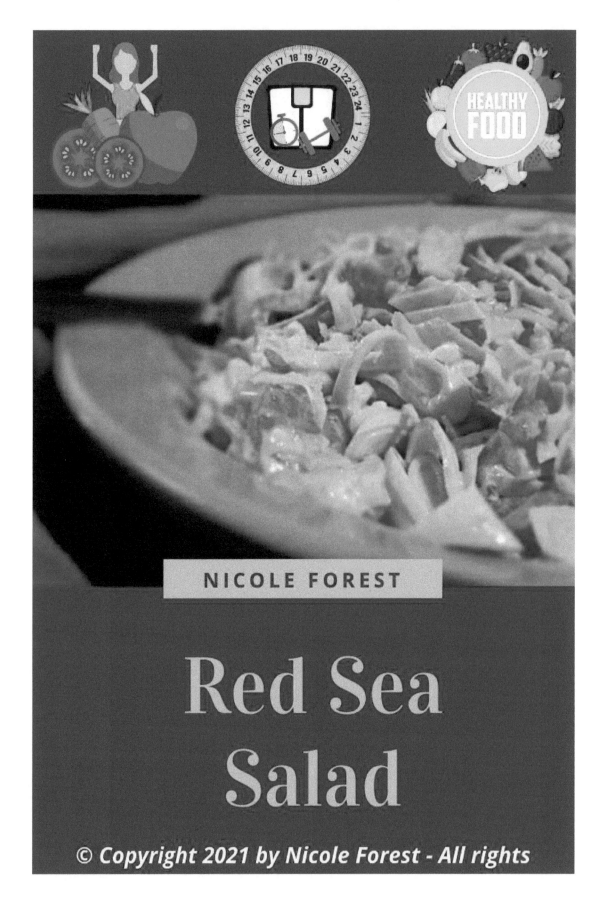

NICOLE FOREST

Red Sea Salad

22. VERY ORIGINAL NEGRESCO SALAD

We need:

-Smoked chicken breast - 350 gr,

-fresh champignons - 300 gr,

- prunes - 200 gr,

- chicken eggs - 6 pcs,
-head onion,

-fresh cucumber,

- olives - several pieces,

-mayonnaise.

Cooking method:

Negresco salad is very similar in appearance to a cake. Undoubtedly, such food will always decorate the festive table. I recommend taking note of the culinary recipe for a holiday salad, for the preparation of which you need a form of any kind. We put the components of the salad in layers, smearing with mayonnaise.

The first layer is smoked chicken breast cut into strips. The
second layer is mashed yolks of 6 eggs.
The third layer is prunes cut into strips (pre-soaked in boiling water for several hours).

The fourth layer - mushrooms fried with onions (sprinkle with salt and pepper).

The fifth layer is a fresh cucumber, chopped into strips (salt).

The sixth layer is smoked breast. Make the top layer as in the photo. The light part is three egg whites, grated on a fine grater.
The dark part is three egg whites, grated on a fine grater and boiled in strong tea for several minutes.

The dividing line is chopped olives.
Negresco salad is ready, bon appetit!

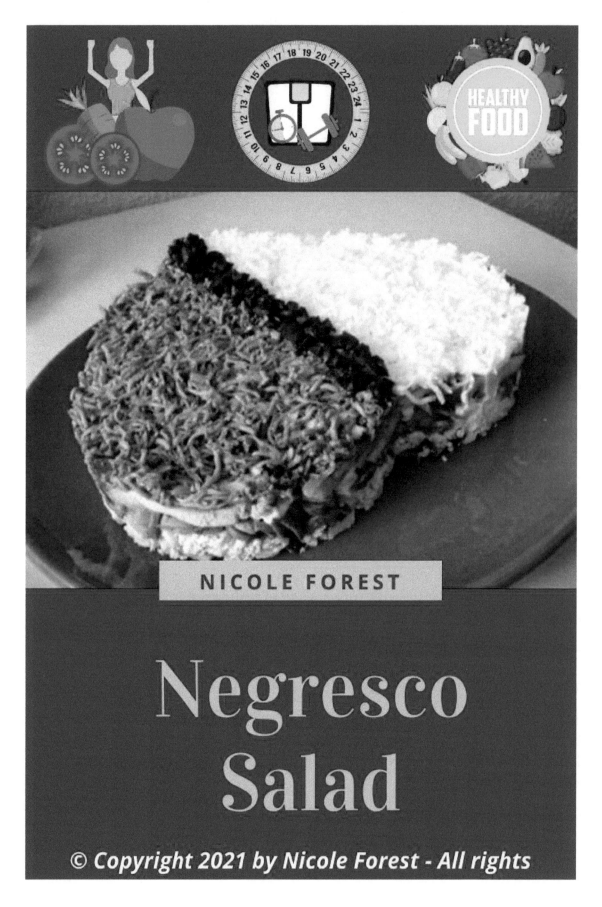

NICOLE FOREST

Negresco Salad

23. "FLAGMAN" SALAD

Ingredients:

Red fish (salted) - 200 gr
Egg - 4 pieces
Cheese - 100 gr

Tomato - 2 pieces

Mayonnaise, pomegranate - to taste
Green onion (for decoration)

Preparation:

Any salted red fish cut into cubes with tomatoes, boil the eggs, separate the proteins, grate on a coarse grater with cheese, grate the yolks on a fine grater, lay out the salad in layers: fish, sprinkle with yolks, tomatoes on top, then

sprinkle with cheese, and sprinkle with protein upwards grated, garnish the salad with pomegranate and onions

Enjoy your meal!

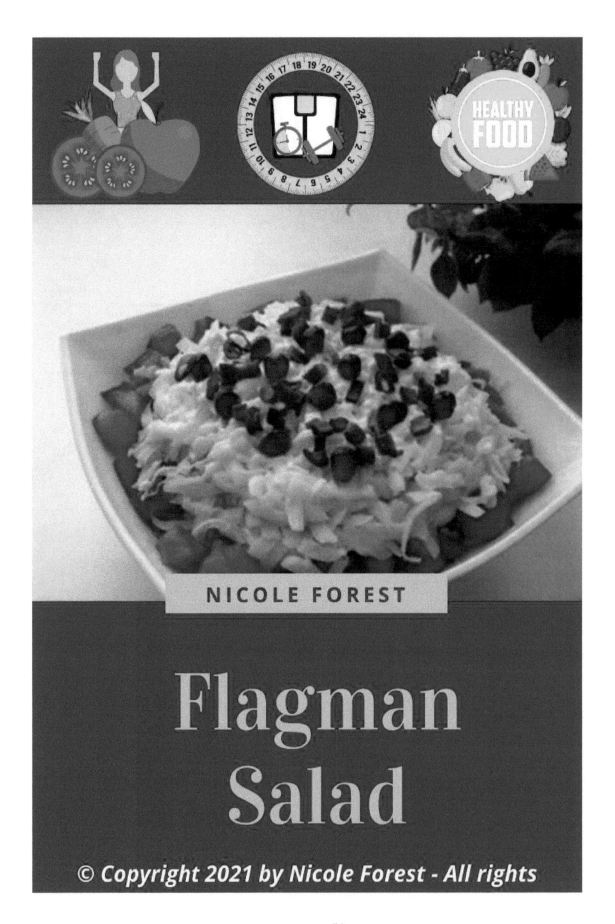

NICOLE FOREST

Flagman Salad

24.   CURD SALAD FOR LOSING WEIGHT.

Ingredients:

Tomato - 2 medium pieces
Bell pepper - 1 small

Greens - to taste, I took half a bunch of dill Salt
to taste
Olives - 1 small handful

Grain curd

Preparation:

1. Finely chop the greens.

2. Cut the bell peppers into small cubes, the tomato into slices, the olives into slices, or you can leave them whole.

3. Mix everything with cottage cheese, salt to taste.

Enjoy your mea

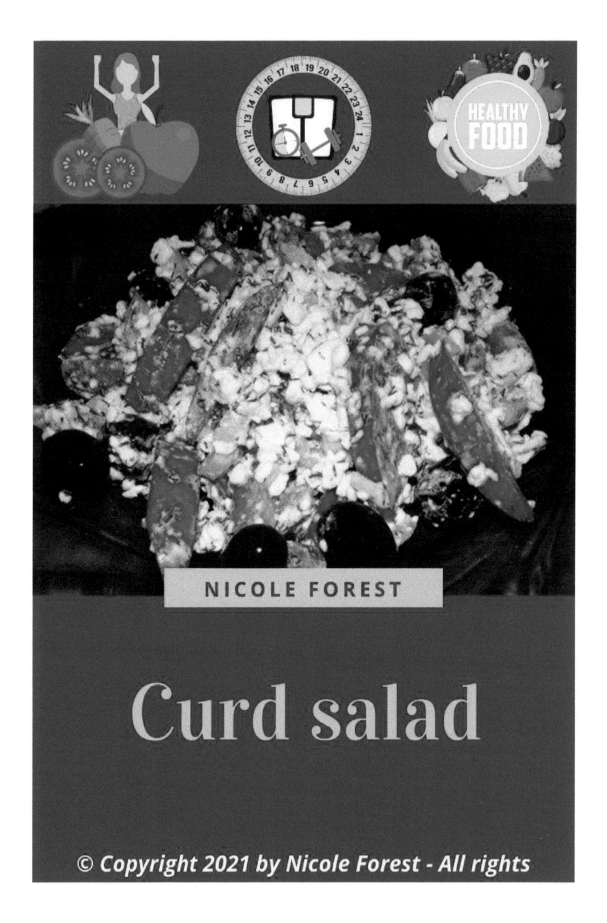

NICOLE FOREST

Curd salad

25. CHICKEN SALAD WITH CARROTS AND GREEN PEAS 250 G OF BOILED CHICKEN MEAT,

100 g canned green peas,
100 gr cucumber
100 g of boiled carrots,

3-4 tablespoons natural yogurt, 1/2
tsp mild mustard
salt.

Dice the chicken, cucumber and carrots. Add green peas, salt and season the natural.
yoghurt

Enjoy your mea

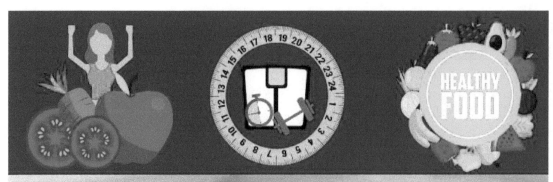

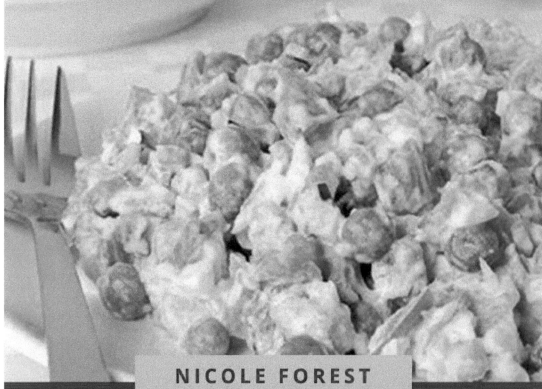

NICOLE FOREST

Chicken Salad

26. DELICIOUS SALAD FOR THE FESTIVE TABLE

Ingredients: Smoked
breast 1/4 Crab
sticks 4pcs
2 eggs

Fresh mushrooms
Cucumber 1 pc Low-
fat sour cream

Preparation:

Boil the eggs and grate (the yolk with the protein separately), fry the mushrooms, finely chop all the ingredients and lay them in layers.

1 smoked breast

2 crab sticks

3 mushrooms

4 protein

5 cucumber

6 yolk

We coat all layers with sour cream!
Enjoy your meal

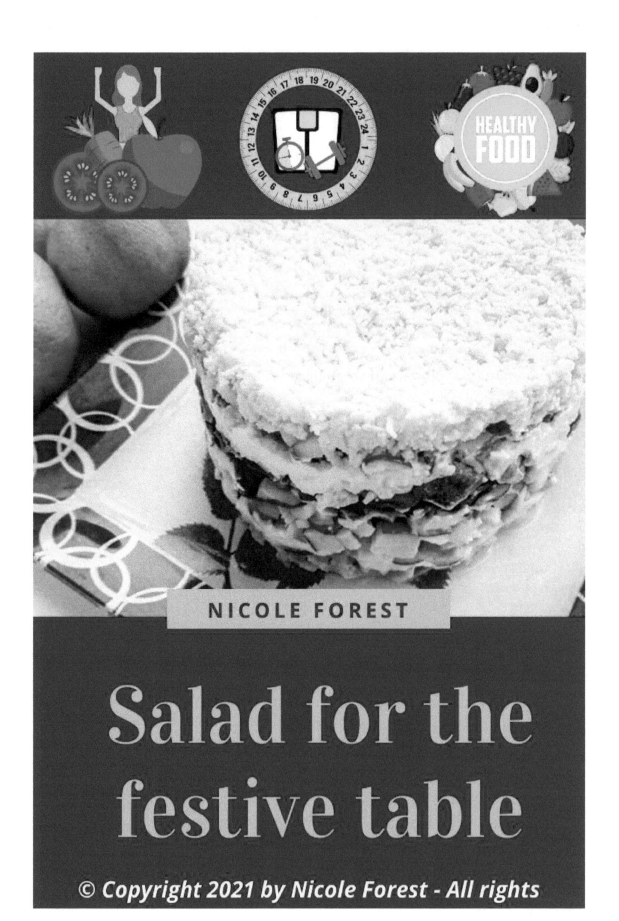

NICOLE FOREST

Salad for the festive table

27. COLESLAW SALAD

Coleslaw is a salad based on the most European cabbage vegetable. It is incredibly popular not only in Europe, but also in the USA, where almost every family has their own version of this salad.

Ingredients:

Red cabbage - 1 small head of cabbage White cabbage - 1 small head of cabbage Carrots - 2 pcs. average
Canned corn - 1 can
Parsley - 1 bunch
Yogurt or sour cream - 100 g

Apple cider vinegar - 1 tbsp. l.
Sugar - 3 tsp
Salt - 0.5 tsp.

Dijon mustard - 1 tbsp l. Ground black pepper - to taste

Cooking process:

1. Finely chop the white cabbage. Mash with your hands. Peel and grate the carrots.

2. Finely chop the red cabbage, removing the hard parts (veins). Mash it well with your hands so that it softens and lets out the juice. Chop the parsley.

3. Drain the liquid from the canned corn.

4. Mix all ingredients. Drizzle with the dressing and mix gently again.

5. Salad dressing: yogurt, salt, sugar, mustard, vinegar, pepper. Mix. Beat a little with a spoon.

6. Let the salad stand in the refrigerator for 2-3 hours, and then serve.

Enjoy your meal!

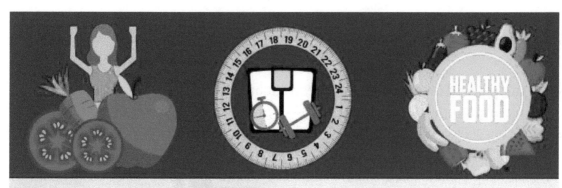

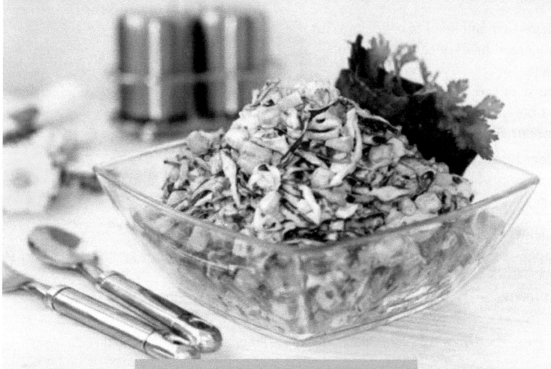

NICOLE FOREST

Coleslaw Salad

28. **FRESH VEGETABLE SALAD WITH BEEF**

Ingredients:

Boiled beef 200 gr. ,
Tomatoes 4 pcs. ,
Red sweet pepper 100 gr. ,

Cucumbers 200 gr.,

Onion 2 heads

Sour cream 10% 100 gr. , Salt,
pepper, herbs - to taste.

Preparation:

Chop tomatoes, cucumbers, red peppers, boiled meat, onions into large strips. Add salt, black pepper, sour cream to taste, mix well. Sprinkle the salad with chopped herbs on top.

Enjoy your meal!

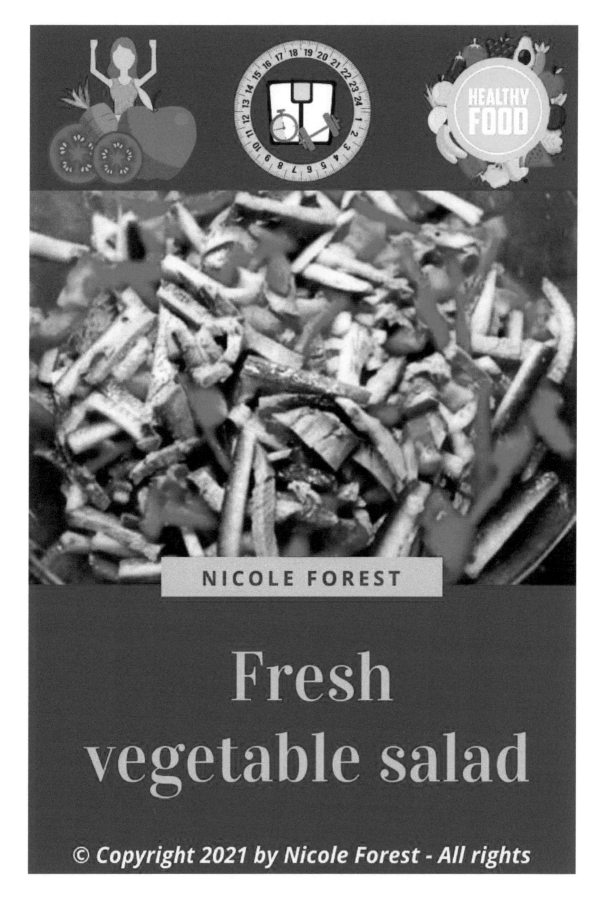

NICOLE FOREST

Fresh vegetable salad

29.   AMAZING CRAB SALAD

Ingredients:

The ratio of ingredients can be any
Crab sticks
Cheese

Green onions A
tomato Yogurt
Squeezed garlic

Preparation:

You can make this salad not in layers, but mix it! Mix yogurt with garlic, chop the sticks and tomato into cubes, grated cheese, chop the herbs! Mix everything or lay it out in layers!

Enjoy your meal

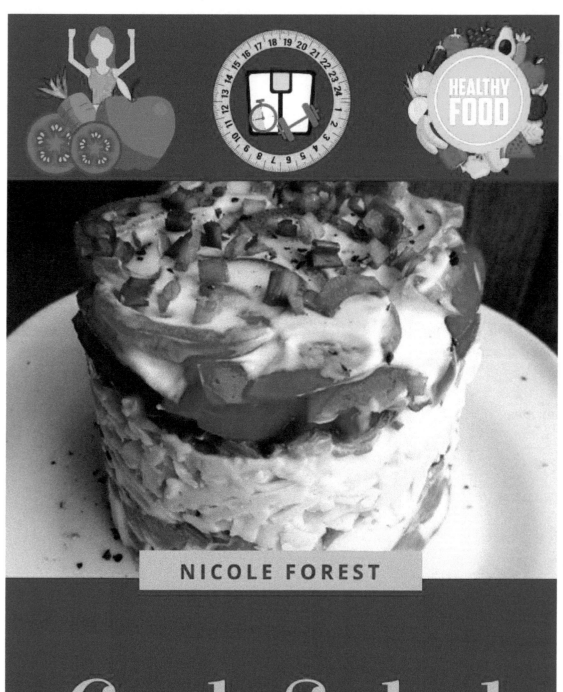

NICOLE FOREST

Crab Salad

30. CHICKEN AND PRUNE SALAD FOR DINNER

Ingredients:

Chicken breast fillet 160-180 g
Prunes 5-6 pcs.
Cucumber 2 pcs. 170 g

Lettuce leaves
Nuts 1-2 tbsp l.
Sweet mustard 0.5 tsp

Lemon juice or vinegar 1 tbsp l.
Honey 1 tsp
Curry (on the tip of a knife)
Olive oil 2 tsp

Salt to taste

Preparation:

Cook chicken fillet. (cool in broth)

Soak prunes in 1 tbsp. l. hot chicken broth Peel
the cucumbers and cut into strips.
Coarsely chop the nuts (walnuts).

Cut the cooled fillet into strips.

Strain the prunes, cut them like chicken.

For the sauce, add mustard, lemon juice, honey, olive oil, curry, salt to the prune infusion.

Beat well with a fork to dissolve the honey.

Put the chicken with prunes and cucumbers in a ring on lettuce leaves. Enjoy your meal!

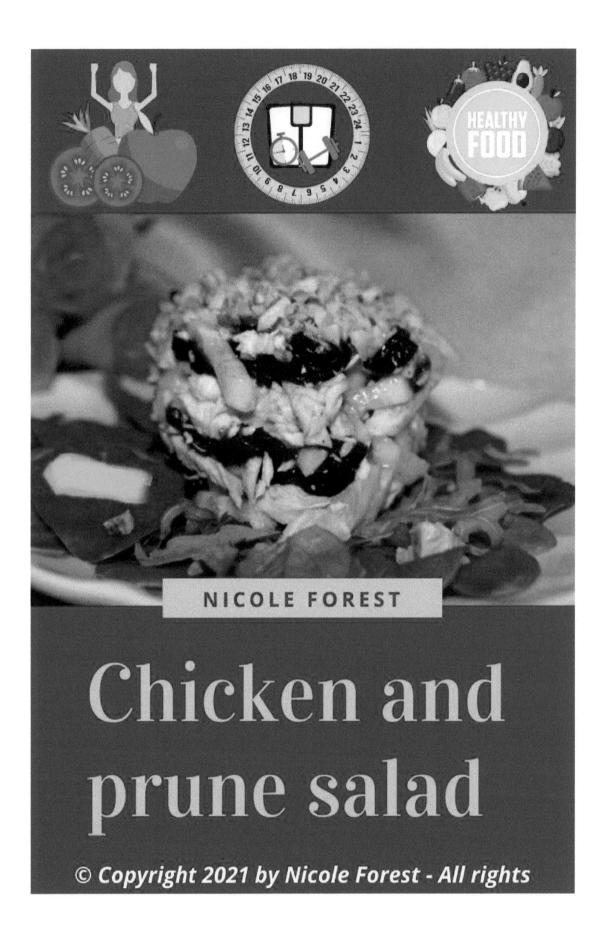

NICOLE FOREST

Chicken and prune salad

31. SALAD WITH CHICKEN BREAST, TOMATOES AND GREEN PEAS.

Chicken breast - 300 gr (boiled)
Tomatoes - 3 pieces
Eggs - 3 pcs (boiled)
Green peas - 0.5 cans
Green onions - small bunch
Salt and spices to taste
Sour cream in half with mayonnaise - for dressing

Cut the chicken breast into small cubes, add the chopped seedless tomatoes, eggs, green onions, peas, salt and spices

Season with sour cream mixed with mayonnaise
Decorate and serve

Enjoy your mea

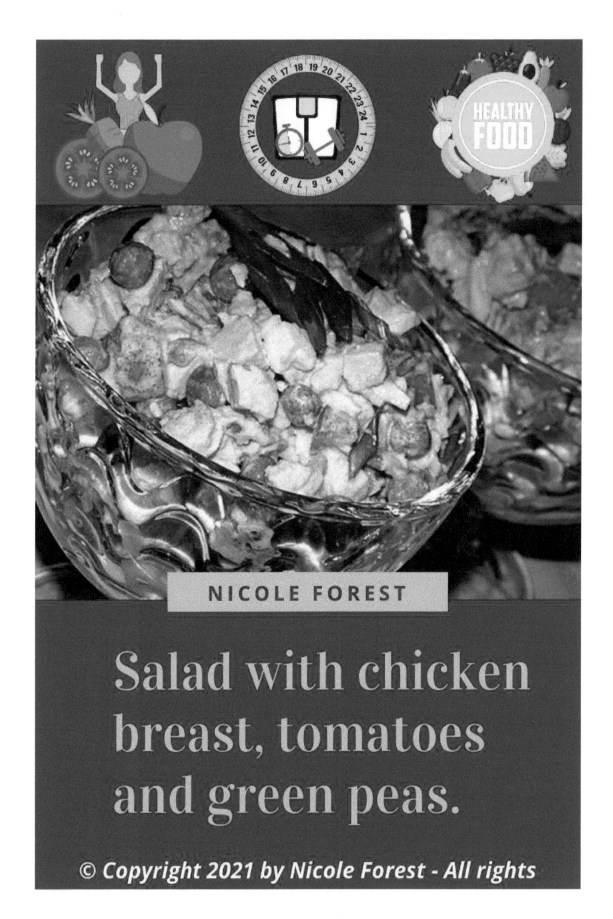

NICOLE FOREST

Salad with chicken breast, tomatoes and green peas.

32. "BRIDE" SALAD.

smoked chicken - 300 g
chicken eggs - 3 pcs.
processed cheese "Druzhba" - 1 pc.
medium-sized potatoes - 1 pc.
bow
mayonnaise

1. The salad will be laid out alternately in layers. There is nothing complicated about this, everything is simple - the main thing is, follow the directions in the recipe.

2. The 1st layer will be finely chopped pieces of smoked chicken.

3. Coat this layer with mayonnaise on top.

4. The second layer in our salad will be pickled onions (to cook it, you will need to finely chop the onion and pour it with a mixture of vinegar and hot boiled water for 10-11 minutes).

5. The third layer of the salad is boiled potatoes, grated on a coarse or fine grater (as you like).

6. Coat this layer with mayonnaise on top.

7. 4th layer consists of finely grated egg yolks.

8. 5th layer - a little processed cheese, grated on a fine grater.

9. Coat this layer with mayonnaise on top.

10. And finally, the top and very last layer is the grated egg whites.

If desired, all layers of lettuce can be repeated again.

Like most flaky salads, the Bride tastes better on the second day, when it is better saturated. You can store this dish in the refrigerator for 4-5 days, but usually it is eaten earlier.

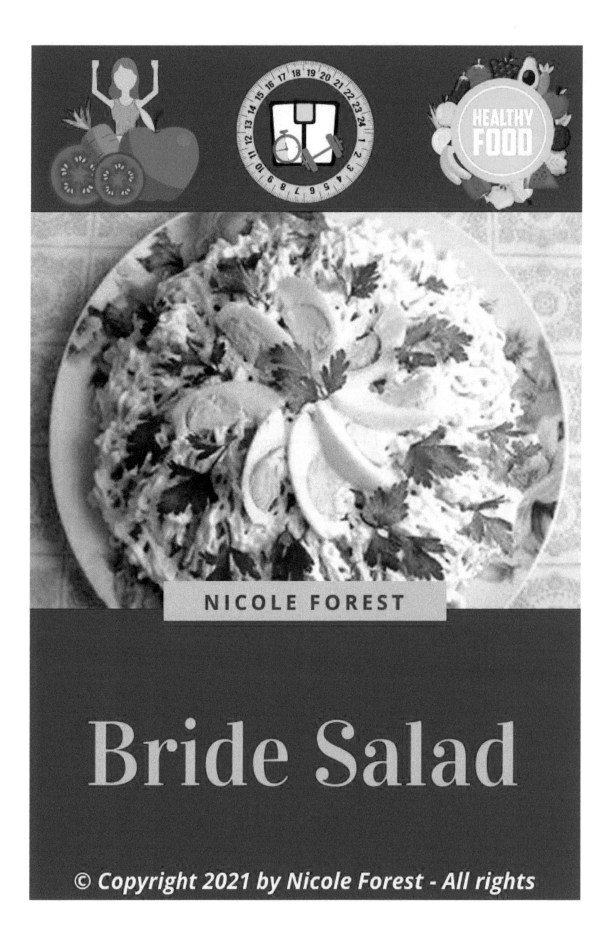

NICOLE FOREST

Bride Salad

33. TOMATO SALAD WITH BOILED SMOKED BRISKET, CHEESE AND CROUTONS.

Fresh tomatoes (hard) - 2-3 pcs; Brisket
(boiled and smoked) - 50-60 g; Hard cheese
- 50 g;
Garlic - 2 teeth;

Parsley - greens (to taste);

Salt, freshly ground black pepper (to taste);
Mayonnaise - 2-3 tbsp.;
White loaf - 2 scrap;

Wash the tomatoes, dry and cut into cubes (the tomatoes must be firm). Also cut the boiled-smoked brisket.

Grate hard cheese and add to the rest of the products.

Salt and pepper the salad to taste, add chopped parsley, garlic, passed through a press and mayonnaise. Stir the salad gently.

Prepare croutons in advance: cut the loaf slices into small cubes or cubes and fry in a dry frying pan until golden brown and crisp. Cool down. Crackers, if desired, can also be used in store (with the aroma of cheese or salami).

Put the salad in a salad bowl, on top - fried croutons. Decorate with a sprig of parsley. That's all, a wonderful and delicious tomato salad with boiled- smoked brisket, cheese and croutons is ready! Serve the salad immediately!

Enjoy your meal!

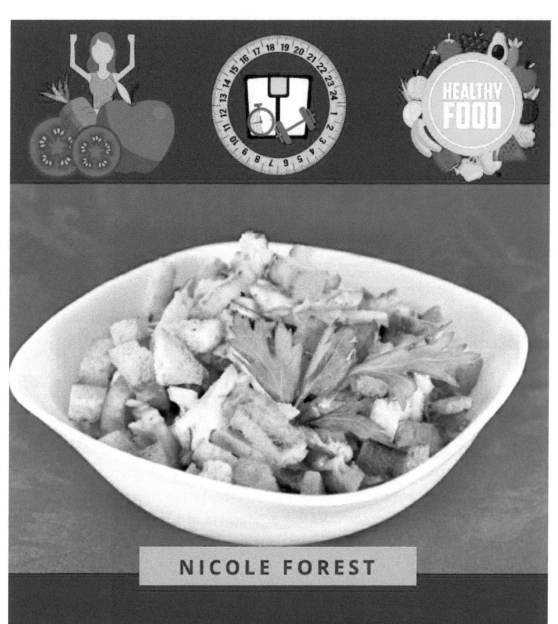

NICOLE FOREST

Tomato salad with boiled smoked brisket, cheese and croutons.

34. FESTIVE COD LIVER SALAD

Ingredients:

- cod liver -1 can (200 g)

- egg - 4 - 5 pcs.

- pickled cucumber - 2 pcs. (salted, pickled)

- canned peas - 0.5 stack.

- potatoes - 3 pcs.

- homemade mayonnaise

- green onion
Preparation:
Grate cucumbers and squeeze lightly. Grate the eggs - separate the white from the yolk, grate the potatoes, finely chop the onion. Drain the cod liver and crush with a fork.

In a salad bowl - lay a bowl in layers: potatoes, cod liver, green onions, mayonnaise (it is more convenient to squeeze out of a bag), cucumber, protein, peas and mayonnaise. Then repeat the layers if there is room left. Sprinkle with yolk on top and decorate as you wish

The salad can be served in layers in a salad bowl or you can combine all the ingredients, season with mayonnaise and serve.

Enjoy your meal

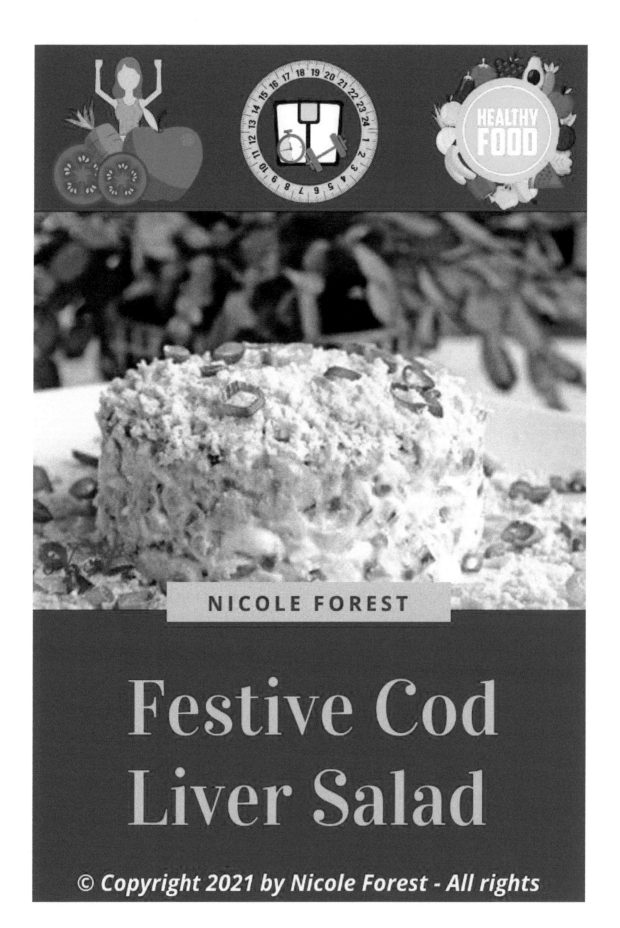

NICOLE FOREST

Festive Cod Liver Salad

35. DELICIOUS SALAD WITH HERRING

Ingredients:

herring fillet - 2 pcs. chopped
walnuts - 1/2 cup
champignons - 300 g boiled
eggs - 3 pcs. onions - 2 heads
carrots - 1 pc.

vegetable oil - 1 tbsp. the spoon dill
greens - 1 bunch
green onions - 1 bunch
mayonnaise - 200 g

Preparation:

Cut herring fillets into small cubes, mix with nuts.

Chop the onions in half rings, grate the carrots on a coarse grater. Combine vegetables, fry in oil, avoiding discoloration.
Boil mushrooms in salted water, cool, cut into slices.

Finely chop the eggs, dill and green onions. Mix onion with dill.

Place the prepared ingredients in a salad bowl in layers in the following order, greasing each layer with mayonnaise: herring with nuts, eggs, vegetables, mushrooms and herbs. When serving, brush the salad with the remaining mayonnaise and sprinkle with chopped herbs.

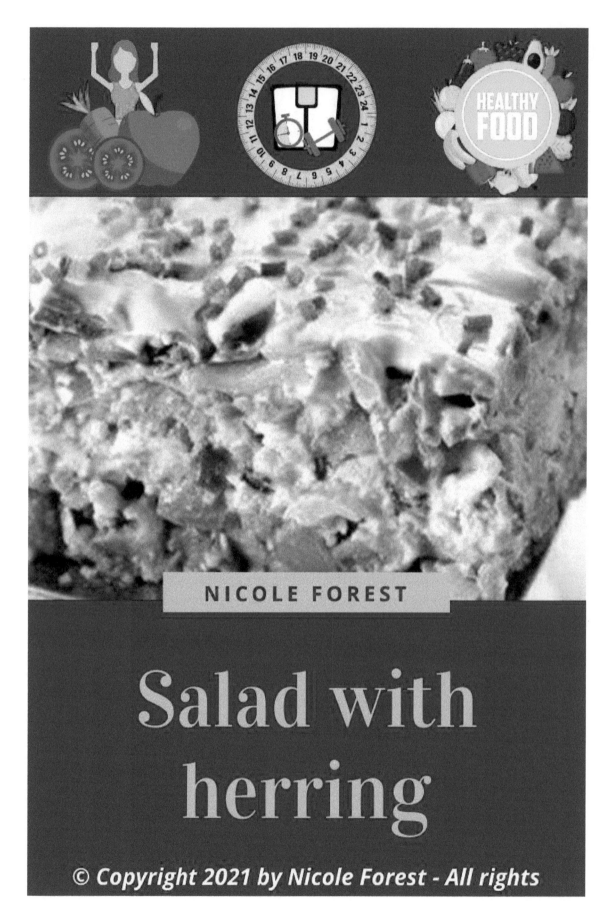

HEALTHY FOOD

NICOLE FOREST

Salad with herring

36. <u>**DELICIOUS VINAIGRETTE**</u>

Ingredients:

Beets - 2 pcs (boiled)
Carrots - 2 pcs (boiled)

Cucumbers - 2 pcs (pickled)
Potatoes - 2 pcs (boiled) Peas -
2 tbsp. l
Salt to taste

Olive oil - 2 tablespoons l

Preparation:

Boil beets, potatoes and carrots. We clean vegetables. Put the pot of water on the stove again. This time for the peas. If you don't have a fresh one, don't replace it with canned, it's best not to add it to your vinaigrette at all. Transfer the peas to boiling water and cook for 7 minutes. During this time, cut the beets into small cubes. We do the same with potatoes and carrots. Chop pickled cucumbers too. We discard the peas in a colander and put them in a bowl with vegetables and cucumbers. Salt, pour in olive oil, mix. If you have enough pungency and "salinity" from pickled cucumbers, you can skip adding salt. It remains to put the salad in the refrigerator, wait until it cools down, and enjoy a delicious dietary meal. That's the whole recipe for a dietary vinaigrette.

Enjoy your meal!

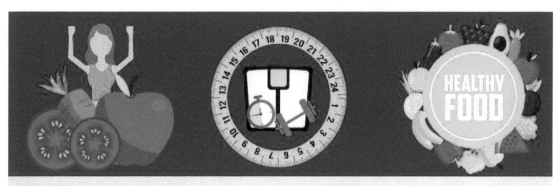

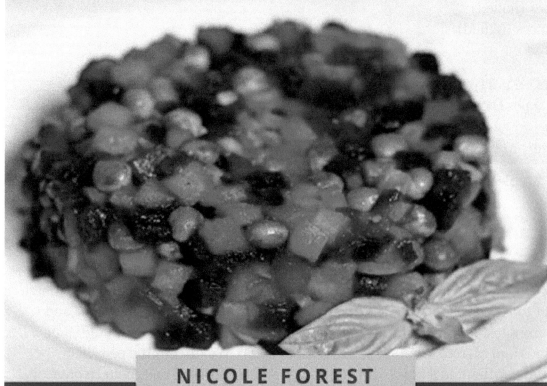

NICOLE FOREST

Vinaigrette

37. **BEAN SALAD FOR DINNER!**

Ingredients:

1 boiled chicken or turkey breast 3
boiled eggs
1 can of canned red beans

1-2 sweet and sour apples
Sour cream

Preparation:

Throw the beans in a colander and rinse well. Cut the chicken and eggs into cubes. Peel and grate the apples. Mix everything and season with sour cream.

Enjoy your meal!

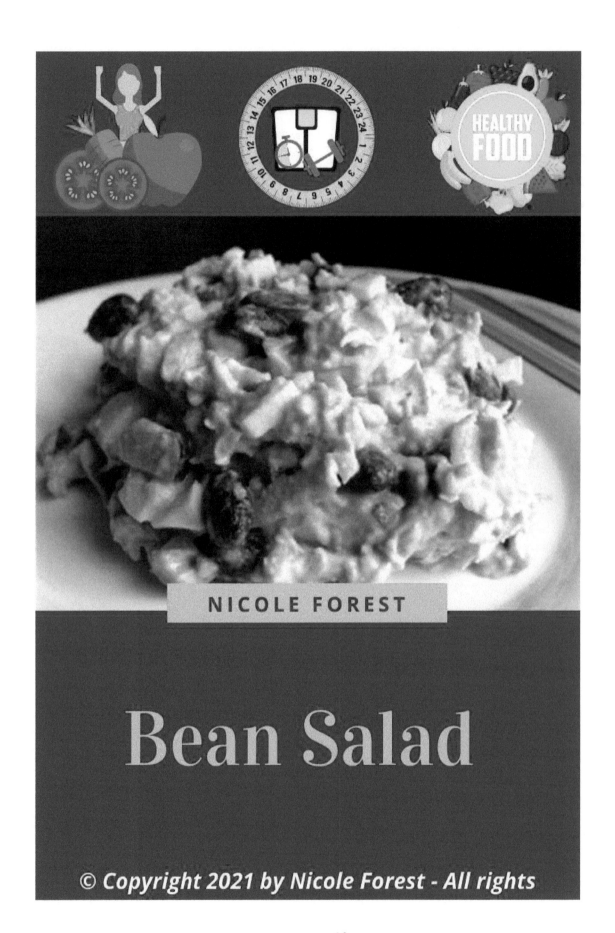

NICOLE FOREST

Bean Salad

38. LOW-CALORIE "PROTEIN" SALAD

Ingredients:

- mushrooms 180gr.

- boiled chicken fillet 2 pcs. (170gr.)

- 1 egg + 2 squirrels

- 2 medium onions (100 gr.)

- cottage cheese 1.8% 100g.

- yogurt 0-1% 100gr.

- garlic 2 cloves

- salt pepper

Preparation:

Boil chicken fillet and chill. Fry the onions in a dry frying pan for 1-2 minutes, add the chopped mushrooms and continue to fry over medium heat (you can over high) so that the mushrooms do not let the water go too much, until golden brown, put on a plate and let cool.

Beat 1 egg and 2 egg whites, add salt and bake a pancake in a dry frying pan, cool and cut into oblong squares. Make a dressing: mix cottage cheese with yogurt, add garlic, salt, pepper.

Cut the chicken fillet into small cubes, add the chilled mushrooms and onions and the protein pancake, cut into pieces. fill the mixture with the ready-made dressing and put it in the refrigerator for a few hours to soak!

Enjoy your meal!

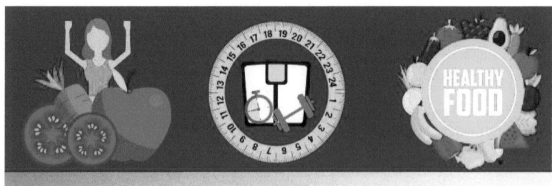

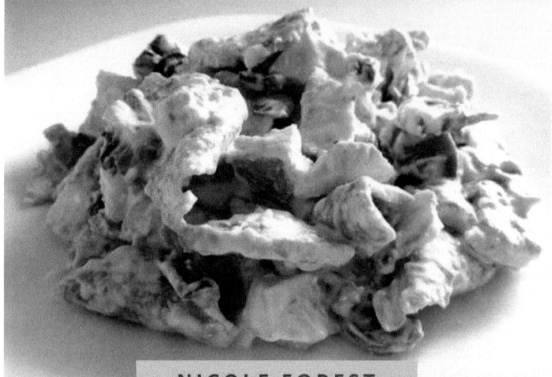

NICOLE FOREST

Low-calorie Protein salad

39.   CHICKEN FILLET SALAD WITH GREEN BEANS

Ingredients:

Chicken fillet - 300 g
Boiled eggs - 2 pcs.
Tomato - 1 piece Green
beans - 300 g Onions - 1
\ 2 pieces Sour cream to
taste Cheese - 100 g
Salt, pepper - to taste

Preparation:

First, boil the chicken breast and eggs. Process the green beans in another saucepan or double boiler. Cut the chicken breast into thin strips, you can also simply divide it into fibers. Cut the cheese, tomato and onion into small pieces. Chop the boiled egg finely too.

Combine all the ingredients in a large bowl and season the salad with sour cream. Stir. Salad ready.

Enjoy your meal!

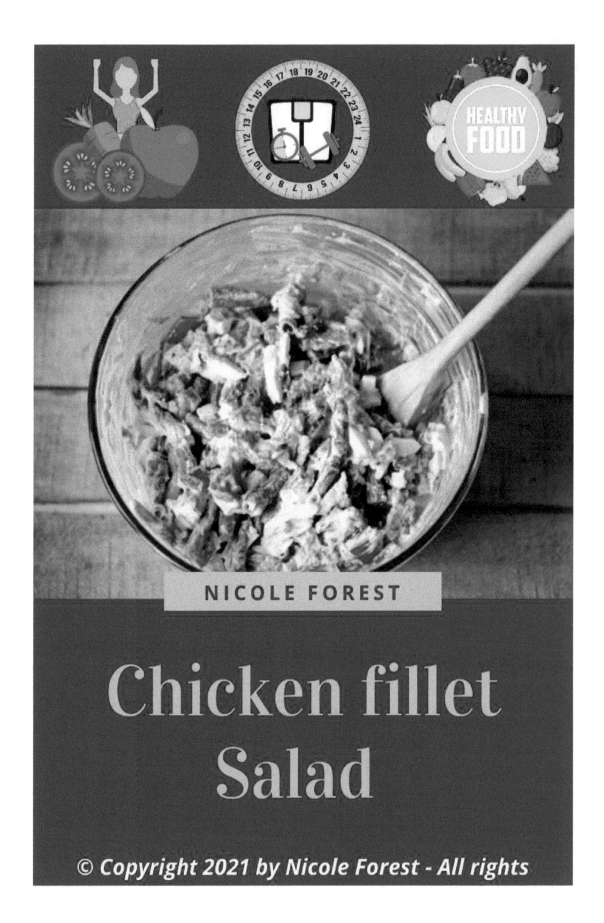

NICOLE FOREST

Chicken fillet Salad

40. **<u>SIMPLE AND HEARTY SALAD</u>**

Ingredients:

- 2 tomatoes,

- 2-3 cloves of garlic,

- 1 can of canned beans in tomato sauce,

- 1 pack of crab sticks,

- salt, pepper to taste

Preparation:

Cut the crab sticks and tomatoes, mix them with the beans (after draining the juice). Chop the garlic finely, add pepper to taste and stir. You don't need any dressings, the salad will be juicy anyway due to the beans in tomato sauce.

Enjoy your meal!

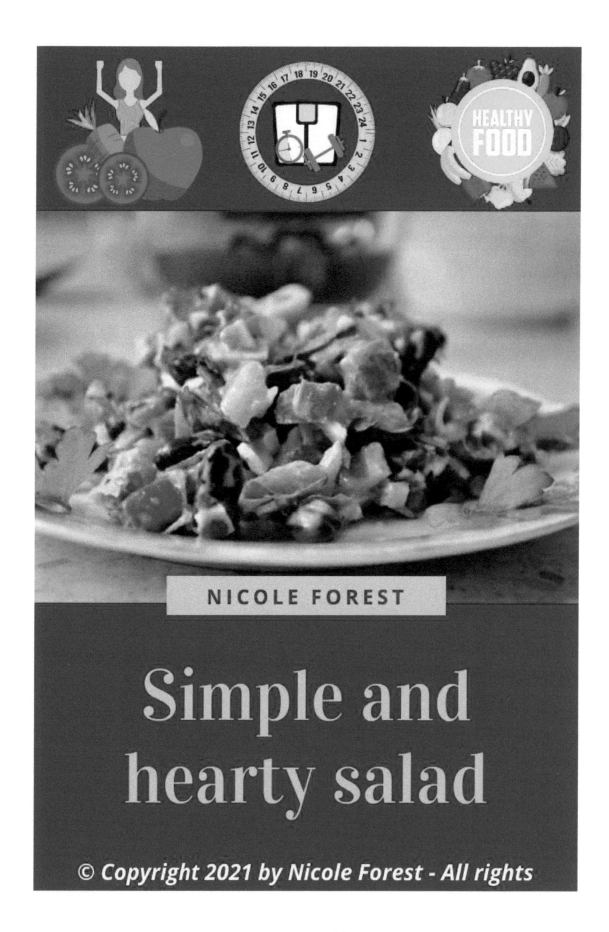

NICOLE FOREST

Simple and hearty salad

41.   CHICKEN BREAST AND CORN SALAD

Ingredients:

2 chicken fillets, about 250 g each 1
medium cucumber
1 large stalk of celery

150 g canned corn (you can freshly boiled in season) sprig
of dill
Salt and pepper to taste

For refueling:

6 tbsp natural yoghurt / sour cream 10% Salt
to taste

Preparation:

Preparing the dressing. take yogurt or sour cream, salt to taste and mix. Set aside.

Cut each chicken fillet in half, lengthwise. Salt and pepper to taste. fry for 2-3 minutes on each side in a dry frying pan (you can use a grill or oven, but time is already according to the situation).

Cut the cucumber and celery into strips

Cut the cooled chicken fillet into small pieces.

Mix the chicken, corn, cucumber and celery, salt to taste and lay out. Water with the dressing and serve. decorate with parsley

Enjoy your meal!

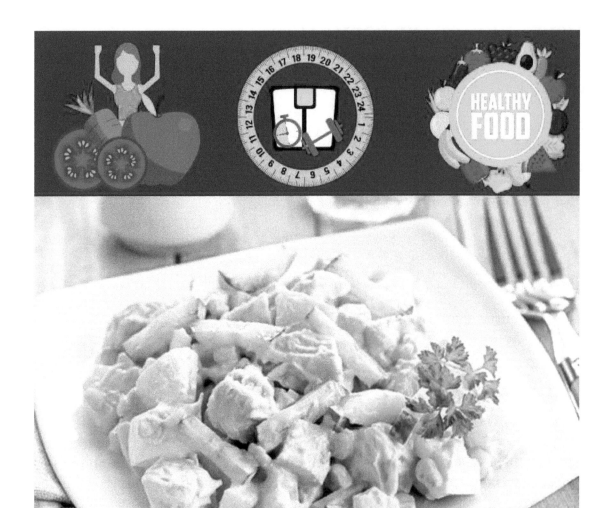

NICOLE FOREST

Chicken breast and corn salad

42.   COLE SLOW DIET SALAD

Ingredients:

White cabbage - 150 g
Apples - 1 piece Celery -
30 g
Carrots - 1 pc

Natural yogurt - 3 tbsp. l
Lemon - 1/2 pc
Salt to taste

Preparation:

Remove the veins from celery, leave the leaves. Cut the celery into thin strips. Chop the celery leaves too. Cut carrots into thin strips or grate. Chop the cabbage. Peel the apple, cut the core, cut into strips. Combine vegetables in a bowl. Add the juice of half a lemon, salt and sweetener to taste. Mix.
Add yogurt and stir again.
Enjoy your mea

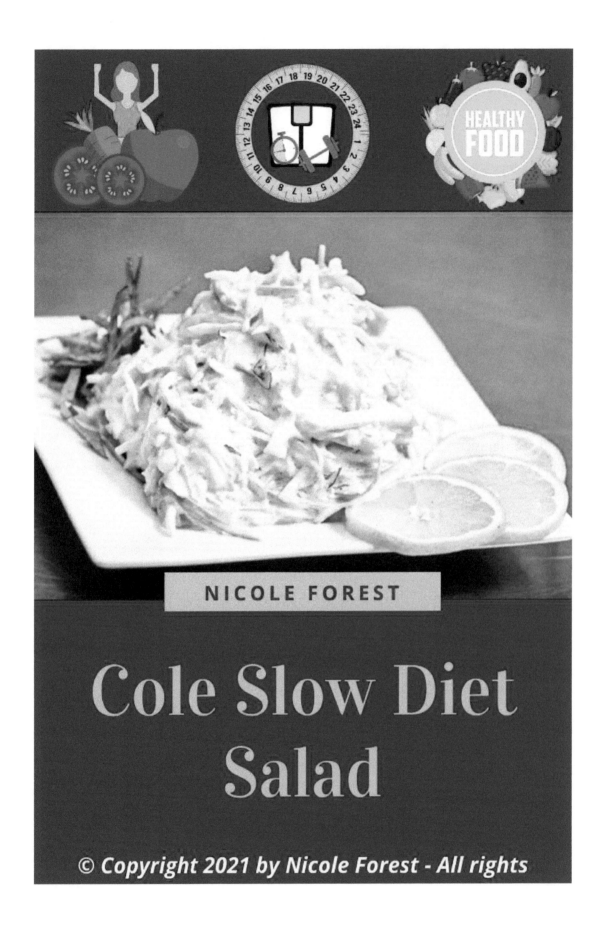

NICOLE FOREST

Cole Slow Diet Salad

43.   FRESH CABBAGE SALAD WITH CHICKEN

Ingredients:
Chicken breast - 500 g
White cabbage - 400 g
Cheese 17% - 150 g
Kefir 0% - 150 ml
Salt to taste

Preparation:

1. Boil the chicken breast.

2. Finely chop the cabbage (without the stalk), put it in a deep bowl and season with salt to taste.

3. After a few minutes, mash the cabbage with your hands to soften it.

4. Cut the chicken into pieces and add to the salad bowl.

5. Add grated cheese and mix everything.

6. Season with kefir and mix again.

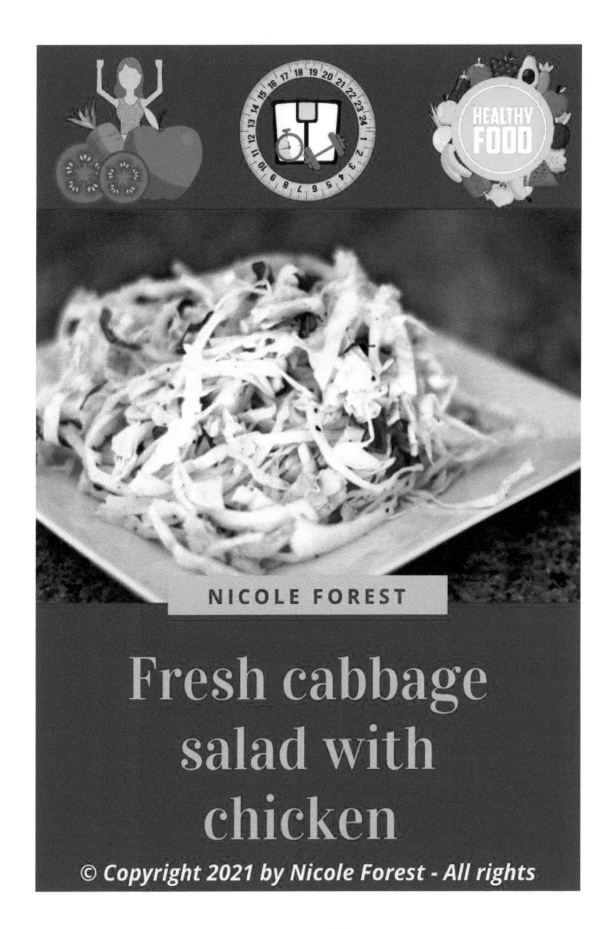

NICOLE FOREST

Fresh cabbage salad with chicken

44. BEETROOT SALAD: THE RIGHT YUMMY!

Ingredients:
Beets - 300 g
Egg - 2 pieces
Cheese - 80 g

Natural yogurt - 3 tbsp l
Garlic to taste
Salt, pepper - to taste

Preparation:

Cut the peeled boiled beets into small cubes, place in a salad bowl. Cut the cheese and peeled eggs into small cubes. Add them to the beetroot salad bowl. Season salad with salt, season with yogurt, season with spices to taste. Stir the salad. Serve immediately after preparation.

Enjoy your meal!

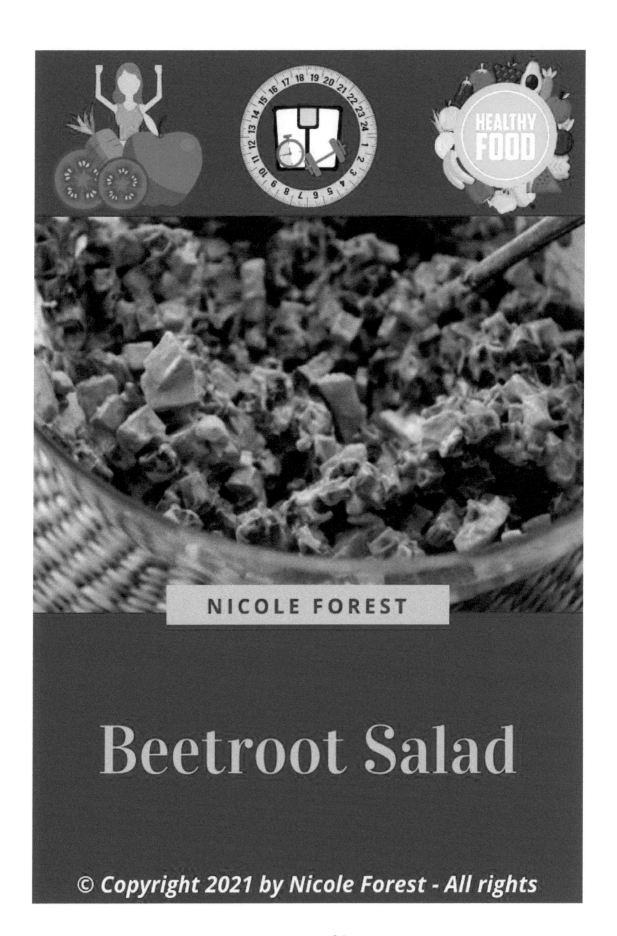

NICOLE FOREST

Beetroot Salad

45. SALAT "EMERALD"

Ingredients:
-Ham - 200 g

-Egg - 3 pieces

-Mushrooms - 150 g

-Cheese (parmesan) - 100 g

-Onion - 1 piece

-Mayonnaise

-Salt

-Cucumber (for decoration) - 2 pieces

Preparation:

Cut the ham into cubes.

Boil eggs, peel and cut into small cubes.

Chop the onion and champignons and fry in a little vegetable oil. Grate cheese.
Mix all ingredients (except cucumbers), salt, season with mayonnaise or sour
cream, mix. Form the salad on a flat plate. Cut thin strips of cucumber and, starting
from the top, clockwise, obliquely, alternately press them into the salad and so on to the
very bottom.

Enjoy your meal!

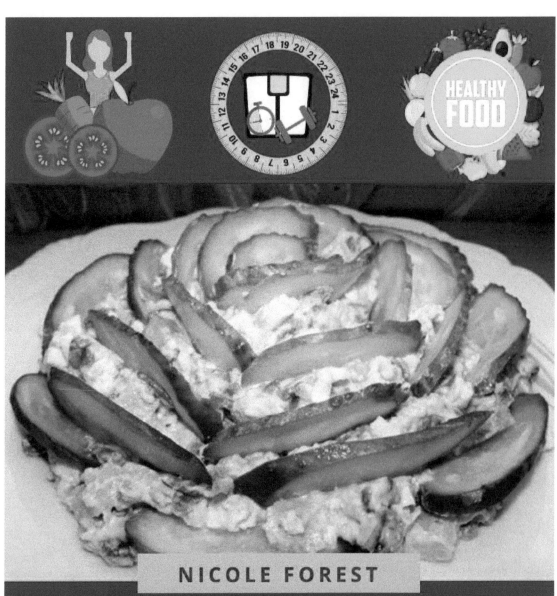

NICOLE FOREST

Salat Emerald

46. BAKED SALMON WITH MUSHROOMS

Ingredients:

450 g salmon fillet

60g fresh spinach, chopped 120
g mushrooms, chopped 1
tomato, finely chopped
1/4 cup olive oil dressing (such as sun-dried tomatoes)

Preparation:

Preheat oven to 190 degrees.

Place the fillets in a greased baking dish.

Combine the rest of the ingredients and place on top of the fillets. Bake for 20-25 minutes until tender.

Salad with chicken fillet, croutons and vegetables
Ingredients:

- 350 g boiled chicken breast

- 2-3 medium tomatoes

- 2-3 medium sweet bell peppers

- 2 medium fresh cucumbers

- 2 packs of rye croutons, 40 g each

- 1 head of garlic

- 150 g of hard cheese

- mayonnaise

Preparation:

1. Either cut the chicken or tear it into small strips. Place on the bottom of the plate or in a salad bowl with sides. Slightly crush.

2. Cut the tomato into small cubes or strips. Pass half the garlic through a press. Combine tomatoes, garlic and a little mayonnaise in a separate plate.

3. Put on top of the chicken fillet. Drain the water from the tomato.

4. Remove seeds from bell pepper and cut into small cubes. Pass the remaining half of the garlic through a press. Mix pepper, garlic and mayonnaise.

5. Put the pepper on top of the tomatoes.

6. Cut the cucumbers into small cubes and lay out in the next layer.

7. Then comes a layer of crackers.

8. Gently grease a layer of croutons with mayonnaise.

9. Grate cheese on a fine grater and sprinkle generously on our salad. Refrigerate for 1 hour.

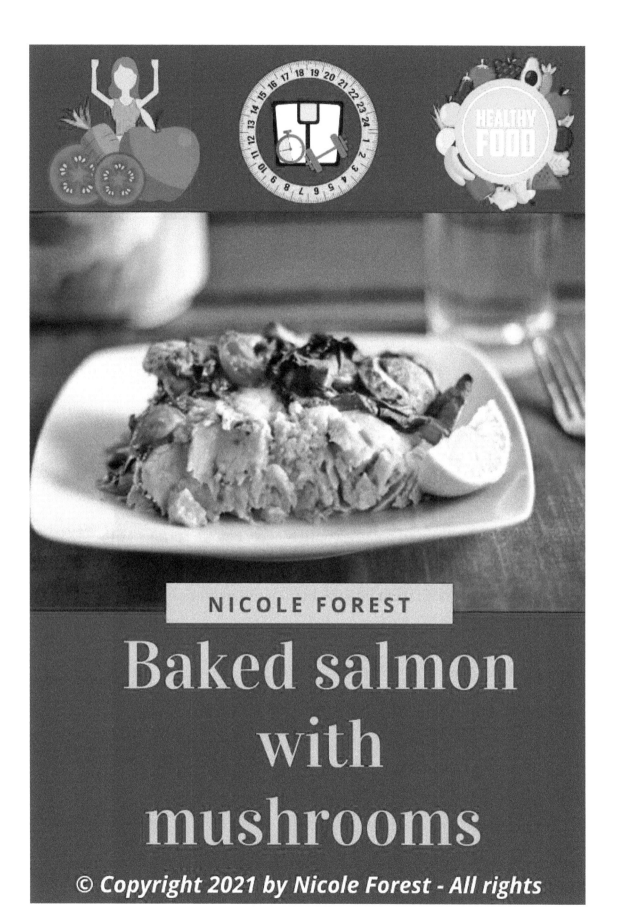

NICOLE FOREST

Baked salmon with mushrooms

47.   VENICE SALAD

Ingredients:

- 400 g chicken breast

- 300 g champignons

- 200 g prunes

- 200 g cheese

- 2-3 potatoes

- 2-3 eggs

- 1 cucumber

- mayonnaise for dressing

Preparation:

1. Pre-boil chicken breast, eggs and potatoes until tender. Pour the prunes with boiling water for 15 minutes. Fry the mushrooms in vegetable oil.

2. Put in a split form in layers, first cut into medium pieces of prunes

3. Then boiled chicken breast, cut into pieces. A layer of mayonnaise.

4. Then diced potatoes. A layer of mayonnaise.

5. Then a layer of fried mushrooms. Do not add mayonnaise after mushrooms!

6. Then a layer of grated eggs on a fine grater goes into the salad. A layer of mayonnaise.

7. The next layer is cheese, grated on a coarse grater.

8. On top of our Venetian salad, grate the cucumber on a medium grater or cut into thin rings. We decorate the salad at our discretion.

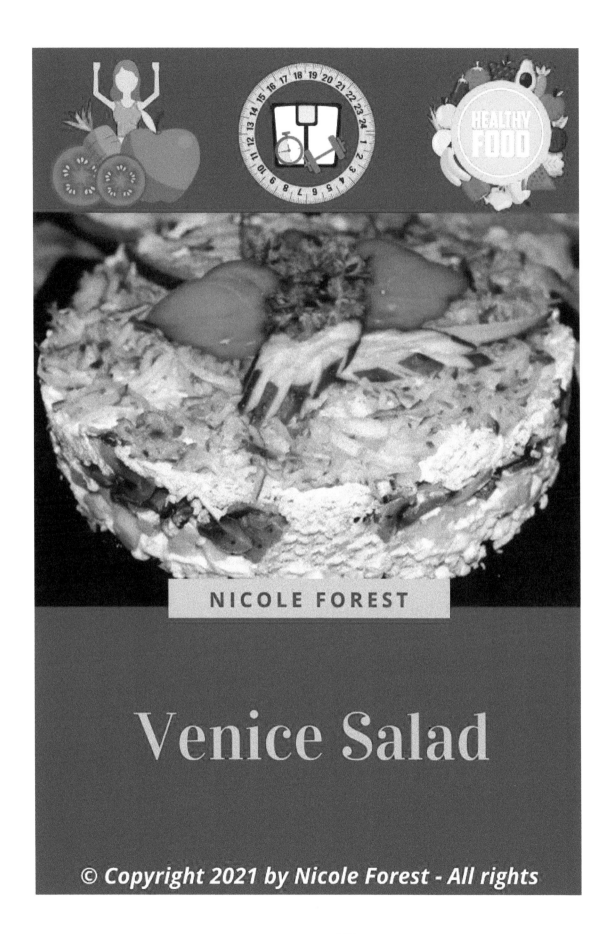

NICOLE FOREST

Venice Salad

48. EGG AND HAM SALAD

You will need:

- 400-500 g smoked ham

- 4 eggs

- 1 sweet pepper

- 1 cucumber

- 1 can (350 g) canned corn

- a small bunch of fresh dill

- mayonnaise

- salt

How to cook:

1. Prepare the ingredients: Hard boil the eggs, wash the bell peppers, cucumber and dill in cold water, drain the corn.

2. Slice eggs into a large bowl. Add corn and stir.

3. Cut the ham into thin, long pieces and add them to a bowl.

4. Cut the peppers into strips. Peel the cucumber, cut it in half lengthwise and cut into thin slices. Add everything to a bowl.

5. Chop fresh dill and add to salad. Mix everything, salt to taste, then add mayonnaise and mix again.

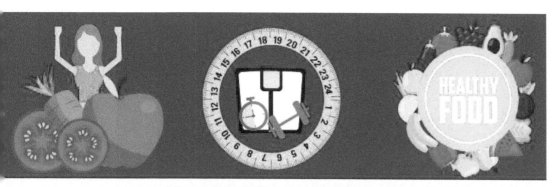

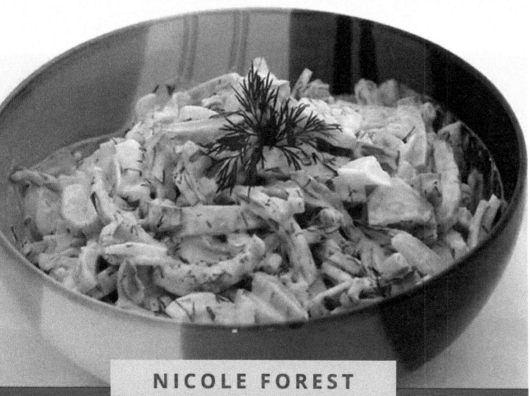

NICOLE FOREST

Egg and ham salad

49. LAYERED SALAD "MY GENERAL"

Ingredients:
100 g hard cheese 4 eggs
2 boiled carrots

2 boiled beets cooked meat
garlic mayonnaise

Preparation:

1st layer: finely chop the meat, add the garlic pressed through the garlic, mayonnaise, mix everything.

2nd layer: grated cheese, mayonnaise.

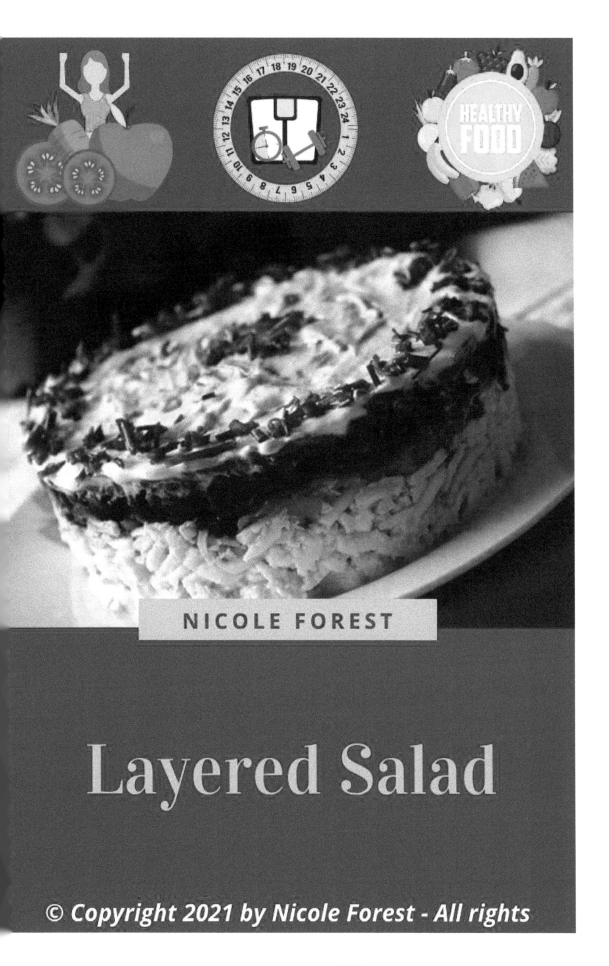

NICOLE FOREST

Layered Salad

FAVORITES

Lightning Source UK Ltd.
Milton Keynes UK
UKHW051118260521
384399UK00003B/153

9 781803 009681